T0261067

Alternative Bypass Conduits and Methods for Surgical Coronary Revascularization

edited by

Ronald K. Grooters, M.D., F.A.C.S.

Iowa Methodist Medical Center
Des Moines, Iowa

and

Hiroshi Nishida, M.D., Ph.D.

The Heart Institute of Japan
and
Tokyo Women's Medical College
Tokyo, Japan

Futura Publishing Company, Inc.
Armonk, NY

Library of Congress Cataloging-in-Publication Data

Alternative bypass conduits and methods for surgical coronary
    revascularization / edited by Ronald K. Grooters and Hiroshi
    Nishida.
        p.   cm.
    Includes bibliographical references and index.
    ISBN 0-87993-577-4
    1. Coronary artery bypass.   2. Myocardial revascularization.
    I. Grooters, Ronald K.   II. Nishida, Hiroshi.
        [DNLM: 1. Coronary Artery Bypass—methods.
    2. Myocardial Revascularization—methods.   WG 169 A466 1994]
    RD598.35.C67A447   1994
    617.4'12—dc20
    DNLM/DLC
    for Library of Congress   93-45757
                                                                   CIP

Copyright 1994
Futura Publishing Company, Inc.

Published by
Futura Publishing Company, Inc.
135 Bedford Road
Armonk, New York 10504-0418

LC #:93-45757
ISBN #:0-87993-577-4

Printed in the United States of America.

This book is printed on acid-free paper.

Acknowledgments

We thank the following people for their valuable help and contributions to this book: Dixie Van Syoc for her efficient secretarial and typing services; Joe Rippetoe for editorial and proofreading assistance; Terry Plummer for his invaluable help with illustrations; the contributing authors for taking precious time to provide chapters with additional expertise; the many physicians and surgeons referenced in the book for their contributions to the published literature; our associate surgeons at our institutions for their constant support. We especially thank our wives and families for their encouragement and sacrifice necessary for us to complete this book.

Ronald K. Grooters, M.D.
Hiroshi Nishida, M.D., Ph.D.

Contributors

Masahiro Endo, M.D., Ph.D. *Professor of Cardiovascular Surgery, The Heart Institute of Japan, Tokyo Women's Medical College, Tokyo, Japan*

Charles T. Everson, M.D., F.A.C.S. *Mills Cardiovascular, Marrero, Louisiana*

Jonathan D. Gates, M.D. *Instructor in Surgery, Harvard Medical School, and Associate Surgeon, Brigham and Women's Hospital, Boston, Massachusetts*

Ronald K. Grooters, M.D., F.A.C.S. *Cochairman of Cardiovascular Surgery and Cardiovascular Research Director, Iowa Methodist Medical Center, Des Moines, Iowa*

K. Craig Kent, M.D., F.A.C.S. *Assistant Professor of Surgery, Harvard Medical School, and Associate Surgeon, Beth Israel Hospital, Boston, Massachusetts*

Hitoshi Koyanagi, M.D., Ph.D. *Chairman and Professor, Department of Cardiovascular Surgery, The Heart Institute of Japan, Tokyo Women's Medical College, Tokyo, Japan*

Noel L. Mills, M.D., F.A.C.S. *Mills Cardiovascular, Marrero, Louisiana*

Hiroshi Nishida, M.D., Ph.D. *Assistant Professor, Department of Cardiovascular Surgery, The Heart Institute of Japan, Tokyo Women's Medical College, Tokyo, Japan*

Pablo Padraza, M.D., F.A.C.S. *President, Milwaukee Heart, S.C., Milwaukee, Wisconsin*

Hisayoshi Suma, M.D., Ph.D. *Chief, Department of Cardiovascular Surgery, Mitsui Memorial Hospital, Tokyo, Japan*

Preface

Today, and more so in the future, cardiovascular surgeons will be challenged by an ever-increasing number of patients with a deficient quantity of conduits or poor-quality conduits available for surgical coronary revascularization. This condition most commonly results from previous usage of the standard conduits, the internal mammary arteries or the saphenous veins. Other clinical cardiac conditions that will be increasingly encountered include the severely atherosclerotic and calcified ascending aorta, most frequently seen in the aged, and the diffusely diseased coronary arteries seen in the diabetic or hypercholesterolemic patient. These three conditions will frequently demand that the surgeon use alternative conduits and/or methods to provide a safe and effective coronary revascularization procedure.

The aim of this book is to assist the surgeon with these less-than-ideal conditions and provide both the new and clinically active surgeon a reference source for the use of alternative conduits and surgical coronary artery revascularization methods reported in the literature or experienced by the contributors. Much of the reported material scattered throughout the literature of the last 20 to 25 years is not only historically important but also useful. Thus, we felt it was time to consolidate this information into a comprehensive guide to meet the challenges of the redo operation involving the calcified ascending aorta or the extensive diffusely atherosclerotic coronary artery.

We realize that it is not possible to provide an exact protocol for all the combinations of alternatives that could be used for these different clinical situations. This book cannot be a "cookbook" since, frequently, there is more than one way to accomplish a coronary revascularization objective. Additionally, the choice of method or conduit often depends on the ability, experience, and preference of each surgeon. Thus, the door for judgment must be left open.

It is our hope that this book may stimulate colleagues to search further for answers through continued research of the many alternative conduits and methods reported. We hope many surgeons take up the challenge and use their imagination to gain new insight that will provide improved short- and long-term benefit. For example, in Chapter 3, usage of the lesser saphenous vein was reported by only three limited studies. Are these studies sufficient? According to Chapter 7, the inferior epigastric artery may have a place in coronary revascularization but how exactly, and when? Chapter 8 suggests that the radial artery may be making a comeback through improved pharmacological intervention, but will this conduit be an effective long-term choice? Could the splenic artery, discussed in Chapter 9, be as good as any venous conduit in some situations? Should the lateral costal artery (Chapter 11) be sought more often for usage? When or how should bilateral internal mammary grafting (Chapter 12) be used to gain revascularization of a greater part of the myocardium? Are composite grafts (Chapter 15) really safe and helpful? Is sequential "snake grafting" (Chapter 17) still an option? And when? Should the alternatives discussed in Chapters 18, 19, and 20 be used before others? Was selective retrograde coronary venous bypass (Chapter 21) abandoned too early as a method? Can the use of a surgical fistula during venous coronary artery grafting (Chapter 22) be helpful? Can the extensive coronary artery endarterectomy (Chapter 24) be improved? Does transluminal angioplasty (balloon or laser) (Chapters 25 and 26) add any value during bypass surgery? Finally, in Chapter 27, will the artificial conduit ever be perfected for the coronary bypass position and approach the standards set by the arterial or venous conduits we use today?

It is an honor for us to contribute this accumulation of ideas and build an armamentarium so that the surgeon will have the readily available information and reference material to gain maximum benefit for the patient with difficult surgical coronary artery presentations. We hope this book will stimulate and inspire surgeons to conceive of other ingenious solutions and, at the same time, provide a concise, practical, and comprehensive guide for situations in which alternative conduits and methods are needed.

Ronald K. Grooters, M.D.
Hiroshi Nishida, M.D., Ph.D.

Contents

Part I
The Standard Conduits

Chapter 1

The Internal Mammary Artery

Ronald K. Grooters and Hiroshi Nishida

The standard bypass conduit of choice for surgical coronary revascularization is without a doubt the internal mammary artery (IMA). Most cardiac surgeons today use at least one of the internal mammary arteries in a majority of their bypass operations, but it did take nearly 30 years for this conduit to be effectively used on a regular basis. A number of surgeons were ahead of their time beginning with Murray et al.[1] in 1954, who first proposed that the IMA would be a usable conduit to prevent the formation of an infarct of the heart secondary to a coronary stenosis. His canine experiments were very successful, demonstrating that it required only a minimum of 20 cc of blood per minute going through the distal coronary artery segment of the IMA bypass to prevent infarction.

It was not until 1961, when Goetz and colleagues[2] used a nonsuture technique with a tantalum ring, that the IMA was first used in human beings as a bypass conduit. On February 25, 1964, the famous Russian surgeon, Kolesov,[3] first performed a left IMA bypass to one of the marginal branches of the circumflex coronary artery using a sutured end-to-end anastomosis similar to Fig. 1. It is interesting to note that he used a "pinch test" to discriminate between a totally obstructed vessel and a narrowed one. If tachycardia or electrocardiographic changes developed as a result of the "pinched artery," it was assumed that the artery, though narrowed, was hemodynamically significant, and a cardiopulmonary bypass was then used to facilitate the operation. Kolesov[4] just recently summarized the results of 32 pa-

From Grooters RK and Nishida H: (editors): *Alternative Bypass Conduits and Methods for Surgical Coronary Revascularization.* © Futura Publishing Co., Inc., Armonk, NY, 1994.

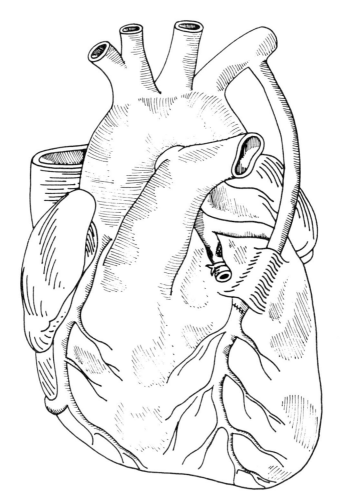

Fig. 1. Drawing of sutured end-to-end anastomosis between the left IMA and the LADA, where the distal portion of the former was tunneled under the epicardium. This operation was performed on a 57-year-old man on January 26, 1965. He lived for 17 years free of angina and died at the age of 74 (from Kolesov VI[4]).

tients he bypassed from 1964 to 1969 and reported that 6 of these patients are still alive more than 20 years later.

By 1968, Green et al.[5] had conducted successful canine experiments in which he used the IMA to bypass a segment of the left anterior descending (LAD). He then proceeded to use the conduit in human situations.[6] Within 3 years, he had operated on 165 patients using the IMA. Angiographic follow-up 2 weeks to 3 years after surgery found only 3% of the IMA grafts closed, whereas 30% of the saphenous vein grafts (SVG) studied in the same group of patients during that time period were not open.

Acceptance and use of the IMA was slow. By 1974, only 5.7% of cardiac surgeons surveyed routinely used the IMA[7] and, in a follow-up survey report in 1980,[8] only 13% accepted the IMA as the graft of preference. Greater difficulty preparing the graft and performing the anastomosis were most likely the significant reasons for its slow acceptance and infrequent use, but flow studies of the IMA graft may also have been the major cause for concern. In 1970, Wakabayashi et al.[9] demonstrated that grafts originating from the ascending aorta had markedly better diastolic flows than did the in situ IMA graft or grafts originating from the descending aorta. In 1975, Flemma et al.[10] showed two to three times the flow in SVGs compared to the flow in IMA grafts. In the 14 patients they studied, they found the diastolic pressure time/tension time index much greater for each SVG. Two years later, Dobrin et al.[11] demonstrated a physiological basis for differences in flow between IMA grafts and SVGs. These conduits were obtained from patients during an operation, mounted in a tissue bath, and pressurized while both diameter and length were measured. Flow velocities were measured for each flow volume and were computed to be three times greater in the IMA than in the saphenous vein (SV). Integration of flow-pressure loss data for the IMA and SV diameters showed that the cumulative pressure loss along the course of the IMA resulted in a greater decrease of exit pressure to perfuse the native coronary vessel when compared with the SV. This provided a quantitative physiological explanation for lower coronary flows with IMA grafting as compared to SV grafting.

Fortunately, others persisted and used the IMA (Table 1). Tector et al.[12] in 1981 reported a 91.6% survival rate of 298 patients at 7 to 9 years postoperatively. Angiographic data demonstrated a patency rate from 0–24 months of 93.4% and at 60–108 months a patency rate of 94.4%, with little evidence of the development of atherosclerosis in the IMA graft. Grondin et al.[13] (Table 1) demonstrated superior angiographic patency of the IMA over the SV and also confirmed that the IMA had minimal atherosclerosis at 10 years. Camerson et al.[14] reported higher survival, fewer myocardial infarctions, fewer reoperations, and a better cumulative event-free survival in 532 patients in whom one or both IMAs were used. The Cleveland Clinic study in 1986 by Loop and associates[15] removed all doubt that it was beneficial

Table 1
Historical Table of Patency and Survival

Author (Date Reported)	Time Period of Study (No. of Patients)	Patency Rate (Time ***)	Vein Survival Rate (Years Post-Op)	One IMA Used: Survival Rate (Years Post-Op)	Double IMA Used: Survival Rate (Years Post-Op)
Kolesov[4] (1991)	1964–69 (33)			18% (20 yrs or more)	
Green[6] (1972)	1968–71 (34)* 1968–71 (84)**	*97% 2 wks–3 yrs **70% 2 wks–3 yrs			
Tector[12] (1981)	1972–74 (298)	*93% 1–24 mo *95% 25–59 mo *94% 60–108 mo			
Grondin[13] (1984)	1972–73 (40)* 1969–73 (238)**	*88.5% 1 yr *84.1% 10 yrs **76.4% 1 yr **52.8% 10 yrs	70% (10 yrs)	84.3% (10 yrs)	
Cameron[14] (1986)	1970–73 (178)** (532)* (38)°*		57% (14 yrs)	72% (14 yrs)	86% (14 yrs)
Loop[15] (1986)	1971–79 (2,306)** (3,625)*		75.9% (10 yrs)	86.6% (10 yrs)	
Johnson[16] (1989)	1972–86 (6,181)		age:<50 78% (10 yrs) age: 50–60 79% (10 yrs) age: 60–70 68% (10 yrs)	92% (10 yrs) 86% (10 yrs) 77% (10 yrs)	60% (15 yrs) 70% (15 yrs) 44% (15 yrs)
Fiore[17] (1989)	1972–75 (100)	R *85% 13 yrs L *82% 13 yrs		59% (13 yrs)	74% (13 yrs)
Galbut[18] (1990)	1972–88 (1,087)	R *84.9% 53 mo L *92.1% 53 mo			80% (10 yrs) 56% (17 yrs)
Gardner[19] (1990)	1980–88 (723)		age: 70 or over 77% (4 yrs)	86% (4 yrs)	

*—IMA grafts; **—vein grafts; ***—length of time from surgery to angiographic study; °*—double IMA grafting; R—right IMA; L—left IMA.

to have at least one IMA used during the coronary revascularization procedure. This ten-year follow-up compared 2,306 patients receiving an IMA graft with or without an SVG to 3,625 patients receiving only an SVG. It revealed a significantly better actuarial survival rate in the group that received an IMA to the LAD than in the group that received only an SVG (Table 1). It was also noted that patients who received only an SVG had 2.00 times the risk of reoperation than patients who received an IMA. Johnson and associates[16] in 1989 reported 10- and 15-year survival rates using the IMA and found no additional benefit with the use of more than one IMA. Their group noted that it was important to bypass the most critical left-sided coronary artery whether it be the LAD, a large diagonal coronary artery, or a large vessel off the circumflex artery. The IMA was not used to revascularize diffusely atherosclerotic vessels. By contrast, both Fiore et al.[17] and Galbut et al.[18] have experienced very good 10-to-17-year survival rates in patients receiving bilateral IMA grafting and feel that improved survival may be significant (Table 1). Gardner et al.[19] just recently concluded that the IMA was beneficial in the aged population greater than 70 years old.

Resistance to Atherosclerosis

The principal characteristic that distinguishes the IMA as the conduit of choice is its resistance to the development of atherosclerosis. Sims[20] reported in 1983 that coronary arteries developed progressive and severe intimal thickening throughout life, but the IMA showed no more than slight changes at any age. He speculated that this freedom from disease strongly suggested that a local or anatomical factor, such as better perivascular lymphatic drainage, might be primarily responsible for the IMA resistance to atherosclerotic changes. The fact that this resistance seems to last the lifetime of the patient is intriguing. Other investigators, Van Son et al.,[21] reported in 1990 that two anatomical factors in the IMA may provide at least part of the answer. After they compared the histopathology of the IMA with the right gastroepiploic artery (RGEA), the inferior epigastric artery (IEA), and the radial artery (RA), the IMA showed a well-formed internal elastic lamina even at an advanced age and a relatively scant presence of smooth muscle cells in the thin-walled media as compared to the other three arteries. These histologic differences were thought to be important reasons for the low susceptibility of the IMA to the development of atherosclerosis.

Other investigators have noted biochemical differences in the IMA. Prostacyclin, a potent vasodilator and inhibitor of platelet function, was found by Chaikhouni et al.[22] to be produced at more than double the rate in the IMA than in the SV. He concluded that these results provided a possible biochemical explanation for the clinically observed better patency rate of IMA grafts. Luscher and colleagues[23] concluded that a substance they called the endothelium-derived relaxing factor (EDRF) may be present as a mediator. They hypothesized that this substance may be present in significantly higher amounts in the IMA as compared to the SV, which may contribute to the higher patency rates among the arterial grafts. To date, the IMA is the obvious and favored graft, but the few existing clues provide only a partial answer to the big question: "Why is the IMA so resistant to the development of atherosclerosis?"

Complications and Problems

Surgical techniques for harvesting the IMA are common knowledge and have been described and illustrated nicely in other publications.[24-26] Most authors agree that an appropriate technique for the preparation of the IMA must meet three requirements: (1) the vessel must be of sufficient length; (2) the dissection or harvest must minimize or eliminate damage to the vessel wall; and (3) early and adequate flow is vitally necessary to assure coronary revascularization. These three requirements, if present, will eliminate most of the direct problems of postoperative occlusion or stenosis of the IMA conduit.

Use of the IMA can influence other technical factors of coronary revascularization such as a prolonged crossclamp time, cardiopulmonary bypass time, operative time, and increased chest tube drainage,[27] but use of the IMA in a group of patients did not affect their operative mortality. Cosgrove et al.[28] have documented a significantly greater incidence of blood transfusion, and Buxton et al.[29] have reported a significantly higher incidence of perioperative myocardial infarction, but these complications also did not increase the operative mortality rate. Sternal wound infections do occur at a significantly greater rate,[30] but mostly when bilateral IMA grafting is used. Devascularization of the sternum was suggested as contributing to an 8.5% incidence of sternal wound infections with bilateral IMA graft usage.[31] This is particularly true in the obese, diabetic patient. Bilateral usage should be used reluctantly in this group of patients.

Increased chest drainage, a higher incidence of pleural effusions in the postoperative period, and more chest tube drainage was found after an IMA grafting.[32] Patients with these complications required thoracentesis, or prolonged chest tube drainage, more often than those patients receiving an SVG only, but this was not considered a frequent cause of pleuropulmonary morbidity. Landymore et al.[33] reviewed 106 patients in which the IMA was used and found that 53% of patients at discharge who required a pleurotomy for harvesting the left IMA had a persistent loss of left-lung volume noted on a chest X ray. If the pleura had not been violated, 95% of the patients had a normal chest X ray. It was his recommendation that, if possible, the pleura should not be opened in order to avoid the possible volume loss of the left lung. Persistent chest wall pain after the harvest of the IMA has been reported to occur in about 23% of patients.[34] Only 4.5% of patients with an SVG experienced chronic chest wall pain. Generally, the pain did not persist for the lifetime of the patient, but these patients may need frequent reassurance or even pain clinic therapy.

Uncommon cases have been reported and merit attention. Schmid[35] reported a case of a parallel branch causing an IMA steal. This was successfully treated with embolization. Myocardial ischemia, caused by a left-subclavian stenosis, has also been noted after IMA grafting.[36,37] This condition can be successfully treated with a carotid-subclavian bypass or a percutaneous dilatation. Even IMA fistulization to lung parenchyma after coronary artery bypass grafting has been reported.[38] The cause of this fistulization was thought to be the direct contact between the dissected IMA pedicle and lung parenchyma.

The incidence of angiographic abnormalities has been studied by Baurer et al. in 459 IMAs.[39] Significant abnormalities were found in 118 (26%) arteries. Common origin with another vessel was identified in 48 (11%) of the 459 arteries, large side branches were noted in 41 (9%) arteries, severe tortuosity was seen in 21 (5%) arteries, an atypical course was identified in 5 (1%) arteries, significant atherosclerotic lesions were seen in 2 (0.4%) arteries, and spasticity of the artery was seen in 1 (0.2%) artery.

These conditions and complications are potentially hazardous and always need to be kept in mind, but they still do not overshadow the short- and long-term benefit of the IMA as a graft to the coronary arteries. The potential of the IMA as a conduit for alternative methods of coronary revascularization is almost always superior to other conduits if the integrity of the IMA is maintained during its harvest and its use. The IMA to this day remains the standard conduit for coronary revascularization.

References

1. Murray G, Porcheron R, Hilario J, Roschlau W. Anastomosis of a systemic artery to the coronary. Can Med Assoc J 1954; 71:594–597.
2. Goetz RH, Rohman M, Haller JD, et al. Internal mammary-coronary artery anastomosis—a nonsuture method employing tantalum rings. J Thorac Cardiovasc Surg 1961; 41:378–386.
3. Kolesov VI. Mammary artery-coronary artery anastomosis as method of treatment for angina pectoris. J Thorac Cardiovasc Surg 1967; 54:535–544.
4. Kolesov VI. Twenty years' results with internal thoracic artery-coronary artery anastomosis. J Thorac Cardiovasc Surg 1991; 101:360–361.
5. Green GE, Stertzer SH, Reppert EH. Coronary arterial bypass grafts. Ann Thorac Surg 1968; 5:443–450.
6. Green GE. Internal mammary artery to coronary artery anastomosis: three years experience with 165 patients. Ann Thorac Surg 1972; 14:260–270.
7. Miller DW, Hessel EA, Winterschield LC, et al. Current practice of coronary artery bypass surgery: results of a national survey. J Thorac Cardiovasc Surg 1977; 73:75–83.
8. Miller DW, Ivey TD, Bailey WW, et al. The practice of coronary artery bypass in 1980. J Thorac Cardiovasc Surg 1981; 81:423–427.
9. Wakabayaski A, Beron E, Lou MA, Mino JY, et al. Physiological basis for the systemic to coronary artery bypass graft. Arch Surg 1970; 100:17–19.
10. Flemma RJ, Singh HM, Tector AJ, Lepley D Jr, et al. Comparative hemodynamic properties of vein and mammary artery in coronary bypass operations. Ann Thorac Surg 1975; 20:619–627.
11. Dobrin P, Canfield T, Moran J, Sullivan H, et al. Coronary artery bypass: the physiological basis for differences in flow with internal mammary artery and saphenous grafts. J Thorac Cardiovasc Surg 1977; 74:445–454.
12. Tector AJ, Schmahl TM, Jansen B, Kallies PA-C, et al. The internal mammary artery graft; its longevity after coronary bypass. JAMA 1981; 246:2181–2183.
13. Grondin CM, Campeau L, Lespirance J, Enjalbert M, et al. Comparison of late changes in internal mammary artery and saphenous vein grafts in two consecutive series of patients 10 years after operation. Circulation 1984; 70(suppl.I):I208–I212.
14. Camerson A, Kemp HG, Green GE. Bypass surgery with the internal mammary artery: the graft of choice. Circulation 1986; 74(suppl.13):30–36.
15. Loop FD, Lytle BW, Cosgrove DM, et al. Influence of the internal-mammary artery graft on 10-year survival and other cardiac events. N Engl J Med 1986; 314:1–6.

16. Johnson WD, Brenowitz JB, Kayser KL. Factors influencing long-term (10 years to 15 years) survival after successful coronary artery bypass operation. Ann Thorac Surg 1989; 48:19–25.
17. Fiore AC, Naumheim KS, Dean P, Kaiser GC, et al. Results of internal thoracic artery grafting over 15 years: single versus double grafts. Ann Thorac Surg 1990; 49:202–209.
18. Galbut DL, Traad EA, Dorman MJ, DeWitt PL, et al. Seventeen year experience with bilateral internal mammary artery grafts. Ann Thorac Surg 1990; 49:188–194.
19. Gardner TJ, Greene PS, Rykiel MF, Baumgartner WA, et al. Routine use of the left internal mammary artery graft in the elderly. Ann Thorac Surg 1990; 49:188–194.
20. Sims FH. A comparison of coronary and internal mammary arteries and implications of the results in the etiology of arteriosclerosis. Am Heart J 1983; 105:560–566.
21. Van Son JAM, Smedts F, Vincet JF, Van Lier HJJ, et al. Comparative anatomic studies of various arterial conduits for myocardial revascularization. J Thorac Cardiovasc Surg 1990; 99:703–707.
22. Chaikhouni A, Crawford FA, Kochel PJ, Olanoff LS, et al. Human internal mammary artery produces more prostacyclin than saphenous vein. J Thorac Cardiovasc Surg 1986; 92:88–91.
23. Luscher TF, Diederich D, Siebenmann R, Lehmann K, et al. Difference between endothelium-dependent relaxation in arterial and in venous coronary bypass grafts. N Engl J Med 1988; 319:462–467.
24. Mill NL, Bringaze WL. Preparation of the internal mammary artery graft: which is the best method? J Thorac Cardiovasc Surgery 1989; 8:73–79.
25. Ochsner JL, Mills NL. Coronary Artery Surgery. Malvern, Pa: Lea & Febiger, 1978.
26. Nachef SAM, Angeline GD. Preparation of the internal mammary artery. Br J Hosp Med 1990; 45:339–342.
27. Sethi GK, Copeland TG, Mority T, Henderson W, et al. Comparison of postoperative complications between saphenous vein and IMA grafts to left anterior descending coronary artery. Ann Thorac Surg 1991; 51:733–738.
28. Cosgrove DM, Lytle BW, Loop FD, Taylor PC, et al. Does bilateral internal mammary artery grafting increase surgical risk. J Thorac Cardiovasc Surg 1988; 95:850–856.
29. Buxton BF, Tatoules J, Mc Neil JJ, Fuller JA. Internal mammary artery grafting: is this a benign procedure? J Cardiovasc Surg 1988; 29:633–638.
30. Kouchoukos NT, Wareing TH, Murphy SF, Pelate C, et al. Risks of bilateral internal mammary artery bypass grafting. Ann Thorac Surg 1990; 9:210–219.
31. Culliford AT, Cunningham JN, Zeff RH, Isom DW, et al. Sternal and costochondral infections following open heart surgery: a review of 2,594 cases. J Thorac Cardiovasc Surg 1976; 72:714–726.
32. Hurlburt D, Myers ML, Lefcoe M, Goldbach M. Pleuropulmonary morbidity: internal thoracic artery versus saphenous vein graft. Ann Thorac Surg 1990; 50:959–964.

33. Landymore RW, Howell F. Pulmonary complications following myocardial revascularization with the internal mammary artery graft. Eur J Cardio-Thorac Surg 1990; 4:156–162.
34. Eng J, Wells FC. Morbidity following coronary artery revascularization with the internal mammary artery. Int J Cardiol 1991; 30:55–59.
35. Schmid C, Heublein B, Reichett S, Borat HG. Steal phenomenon caused by a parallel branch of the internal mammary artery. Ann Thorac Surg 1990; 50:463–464.
36. Grande K, Van Meter CH, White CJ, Ochner JL, et al. Myocardial ischemia caused by postoperative malfunction of a patent internal mammary coronary arterial graft. J Vasc Surg 1990; 11:659–664.
37. Olsen CO, Dunton RF, Maggs PR, Lakey SJ. Review of coronary-subclavian steal following internal mammary artery-coronary artery bypass surgery. Ann Thorac Surg 1988; 46:675–678.
38. Blanche C, Eigler N, Barrey CN. Internal mammary artery to lung parenchyma fistula after aortocoronary bypass grafting. Ann Thorac Surg 1991; 52:141–142.
39. Bauer EP, Bino MC, von Segesser AL, Turina MI. Internal mammary artery anomalies. Thorac Cardiovasc Surg 1990; 38:312–315.

Chapter 2

The Greater Saphenous Vein

Ronald K. Grooters and Hiroshi Nishida

The saphenous vein (SV) was first used for coronary artery revascularization by Sabiston[1] in 1962. The patient had a stroke two days after surgery and died. Then, in 1964, Garrett et al.[2] reported the first successful coronary artery bypass, still patent 7 years after surgery. Once Favaloro[3] popularized the operation in 1968 and Johnson et al.[4] used it for multivessel coronary artery disease, coronary revascularization using the SV rapidly became routine and frequent. When Bartley et al.[5] demonstrated the conduit's versatility by using it for multiple sequential bypasses in 1972, surgeons remained enthusiastic. The vein was abundant in quantity, easy to handle, and had superior flow rates when compared to the internal mammary artery (IMA).[6,7] These features, along with the fact that the SV was easy to remove (harvest), may have contributed to the reduced use of the IMA. Yet, after several years, it became apparent that the SV first-year occlusion rates of 12–20%[8,9] and the annual closure rate of 2–4% during the first 4–5 years[10] were inferior when compared to the IMA. By the late 1970s and early 1980s, it was noted that the yearly occlusion rates doubled to 4–8% between the fifth and tenth year postoperatively, and approximately 50% of the grafts were occluded by severe atherosclerotic changes at 10 years.[11] The saphenous vein graft (SVG) had been beneficial to many patients but still had not been a complete success, with only 39.5% of the grafts in satisfactory condition 11 years after surgery.[12]

From Grooters RK and Nishida H: (editors): *Alternative Bypass Conduits and Methods for Surgical Coronary Revascularization.* © Futura Publishing Co., Inc., Armonk, NY, 1994.

The SV is preferred by some surgeons in emergency situations, in patients with poor ventricular function, and in aged patients, but most surgeons agree that its exclusive use has diminished and now must be accompanied as much as possible with IMA usage. In part, the short- and long-term patency problems of the SV may be related, particularly in the sixth and seventh decades of life, to the fact that as much as 95% of the SV has preexisting phlebosclerosis.[13] Hypertrophy of the muscle layer is also noted.[14] Add ischemic and/or mechanical injury during the harvest of the SV, which by its very nature is prone to acute thrombosis, and one can easily understand why the early vein graft occlusion rate is 12%–20%.

Early Graft Closure

Cox et al.[15] summarized the structural differences between the vein and the artery (Table 1). Of these, the extremely vulnerable endothelium is the most important layer of the conduit that prevents early graft closure.[16] This layer is not just a passive lining but rather is active and provides vital functions that maintain the integrity of

	Table 1 **Anatomy**	
	Vein	*Artery*
endothelial cells	larger, thinner; less firmly anchored to subendothelium	smaller, thicker; more firmly anchored to subendothelium
tunica intima	more permeable	less permeable
internal elastic membrane	poorly defined	well-defined
media	thin	thick
elastic lamellar	absent	present
medial smooth muscle cells	few; circular and longitudinal arrangement; widely separated by collagen	circular arrangement; orderly array with collagen elastic fibers, and matrix
vasa vasorum	more anastomoses	less anastomoses
valves	present	absent

the SVG as a conduit for blood. Anticoagulation, procoagulation, immune function, vasorelaxation, and vasoconstriction (Table 2) are all necessary if the vein is to function properly.[17] These functions, when preserved and in balance, may not only prevent early thrombosis but could also inhibit the later development of fibrointimal hyperplasia (FIH) and atherosclerosis. Biophysical [18] and biochemical properties[19] of normal veins and arteries are also markedly different (Table 3). Of these properties, it also may be the diminished prostacyclin (PGI$_2$) production[20,21] in vein tissue compared to arterial tissue that promotes both increased platelet aggregation[22] and intimal fibrin deposition,[23] which contribute to the increased tendency of the SVG to thrombose.

The mediators of both early graft injury are many (Table 4) and are likely causes of endothelial cell injury.[15] To minimize this injury and assure graft resistance to acute thrombosis as much as possible in

---

Table 2
Endothelial-Derived Factors and Vascular Responses

Anticoagulation	prostacyclin
	tissue plasminogen activator
	glycosaminoglycans
	thrombomodulin
	proteins S and C
	EDRF (NO)
Procoagulation	tissue factor
	plasminogen activator inhibitor
	factor V
	platelet-activating factor
	factors V and XII activators
	von Willebrand factor
	fibronectin
	factor IX: a binding protein
Immune function	ICAM-1 and ICAM-2
	ELAM-1
	IL-1
	IL-8
	class I and II MHC antigens
	colony stimulating factors
Vasorelaxation	nitric oxide (NO)
	other EDRFs
Vasoconstriction	endotheliums

EDRF—endothelium derived relaxation factor; NO—nitric oxide; ICAM—intercellular adhesion molecule; ELAM—endothelial leukocyte adhesion molecule; IL—interleukin; MHC—major histocompatibility complex

Table 3
Physiology

	Vein	Artery
elasticity	relatively inelastic at arterial pressures	elastic at arterial pressures
role of collagen	inconsequential	important
lipolysis	slower	more rapid
lipid uptake	rapid	slow
lipid synthesis	more active	less active
PGI$_z$ production	less	more
endothelium	similarity to SMC contraction	inhibitory to SMC contraction
vasoconstrictors	more sensitive	less sensitive
vasodilators	less sensitive	more sensitive

SMC—smooth muscle cell

the early postoperative period, good graft preparation is invaluable and should include the following principles.

(1) Meticulous dissection to avoid crushing or stretching of the graft.

(2) Gentle distention using papaverine[24] and a pressure-limiting device[25] to prevent endothelial cell rupture.

Table 4
Mediators of Early Graft Injury or Closure

Damage during harvesting
    —Direct mechanical trauma
    —Disruption of vasa vasorum
Damage during preparation
    —Exposure to media of low oncotic pressure
    —Hypothermic storage
    —Prolonged distention
Surgical technique
    —Eversion/compression of vessel by sutures
    —Coronary atherosclerosis at the anastomosis
    —Inadequate distal runoff
    —Dissection of distal anastomosis
Other
    —Activation of platelets and leukocytes by bypass pump
    —Discrepancy in diameters of vein graft and artery at anastomotic site
    —Acute exposure of vein graft to arterial pressures

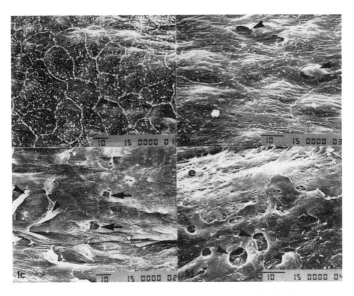

Fig. 1. Scanning electron micrographs. (1a; upper left) Saphenous vein preserved with heparinized blood for 1 hour at 4°C. Normal-appearing endothelium with distinct outline of endothelial cell margins and prominent microvilli. (1b: upper right) Saphenous vein preserved as described in 1a. Minimal endothelial alterations indicated by slight condensation of endothelial cell cytoplasm (see arrowheads). (1c: lower left) Desquamation of endothelial cells (see arrowheads) and pitting or crater formation (see arrowheads) in a vein preserved with the patient's own blood at 4°C. (1d: lower right) Frank erosion (e) of endothelial lining and exposure of underlying subendothelial components in a vein preserved with saline at room temperature. Remaining endothelial cells exhibit severe crater formation (see arrowheads). Original magnifications: 1a and 1c, × 1000; 1b and 1d, × 1500. (from Barner HB[26]).

(3) Use of blood rather than crystalloid solutions of low oncotic pressure[26,31] to maintain the viability of endothelial cells (Fig. 1).

(4) Avoidance of prolonged hypothermic storage, which may cause endothelial cell detachment[27] and impair the cell's capacity to produce PGI_z.[28]

(5) Use of antiplatelet drugs (aspirin and/or dipyridamole) to improve short- and long-term graft patency.[29,30]

Wound Complications and Prevention

The long continuous incision for removal of the greater SV is the standard method to expose and harvest the conduit. Techniques that preserve the vein from intimal disruption and prevent early or late closure are important,[25] but major complications of the large wound such as skin loss or purulent infections result in significant morbidity for approximately 1% of patients[31] and frequently cause a prolonged hospitalization. Minor complications, such as saphenous nerve damage, hematomas, prolonged lymphatic drainage, fat necrosis with cellulitis, and chronic edema, can occur at rates as high as 20%[32] and be very bothersome to the patient and surgeon. The following guidelines and techniques that we use have noticeably reduced vein-harvesting complications.

(1) Obesity, diabetes mellitus, severe peripheral artery disease, and preexisting venous stasis changes must take on significant importance in the surgeon's mind. If possible, avoid making incisions in areas of skin changes associated with venous or arterial disease. If the thigh is obese, veins should be taken, when possible, from the lower leg.

(2) Once a small segment of the vein has been exposed, tracking the direction of the vein using scissors to tunnel on top of the vein before a larger incision is made facilitates staying on a path with the vein. This may prevent the development of large skin flaps that could then lose their blood supply and cause a tissue slough.

(3) Closure of the leg wound is not done until the heparin has been reversed. Following this rule is particularly important for the thigh incision and has reduced hematoma formation.

(4) The incision over the vein is made with a knife or scissors. Cautery is used only for pinpoint hemostasis. Thus, tissue viability is preserved, and wound infections are kept below 1%.

(5) For the patient with obese lower extremities, very meticulous closure of tissues with interrupted absorbable sutures is absolute. Any loose tissue is debrided and/or wiped from the wound. This will help reduce the cellulitis produced by fat necrosis.

(6) All patients are instructed to elevate the leg with the incision above the heart at least 6 inches, 3 times a day, for 30 minutes each time. Patients are instructed to continue the elevation for at least 3 weeks after surgery. Elevation of the leg keeps edema at a minimum. Elastic hose or wraps are not used after the first 24 hours because they tend to constrict the leg above the wound and may cause more swelling. Also, the wounds can be more easily watched without these wraps.

(7) Below the knee, the saphenous nerve and its branches frequently cross over the vein anteriorly. Damage to this structure can

only be prevented by alert and meticulous dissection, which involves staying close to the vein and taking care not to divide the branches as they cross the vein. Upon closure of the wound, care must be taken not to incorporate this nerve tissue into the closure with the sutures.

Late Graft Closure

Fibrointimal hyperplasia (FIH) is histologically described as a relative decrease of intimal cellularity accompanied by a replacement of medial smooth muscle cells by fibrous tissue and increased matrix formation. These changes are seen as early as 1 month after surgery and are the predominant abnormality of vein grafts (VG) in the one- to five-year period postoperatively. As the fibrosis develops, there is a loss of elastic fibers and an increase of the adventitia. This results in a stiff, fibrouslike conduit. By one year, the lumen has decreased by 25%.[30] Although present in nearly all patients studied at 1 year, FIH does not seem to measurably affect graft patency during the first few months or up to 3 years after surgery.[8] This does not mean that surgeons should disregard this potentially hazardous pathological change. Though infrequent, FIH is still responsible for most graft failures within 1 month to 1 year after the revascularization procedure.[9] The etiology of this condition may, in part, be a natural response to the stress of arterial pressures, but it may also be a result of a reparative process initiated by ischemic and/or hemodynamically induced damage.[17,33]

It has been shown that precautions taken to preserve the vein and prevent ischemia do not stop the initiation of intimal hyperplasia but may prevent an exuberant FIH.[34] Of the nine mechanical deformations and stresses to which veins are susceptible when exposed to arterial pressure, low flow velocity may be the likely cause of exuberant FIH.[35] VGs that carry low flow volume appear to develop more FIH than those that carry high flow volume. Coronary vein grafts with flow rates of 60 mL/min exhibit more FIH than do femoral-popliteal grafts with flow rates of 90–100 mL/min.[36,37] In another study of 51 grafts 7 to 100 months postoperatively,[38] FIH was most closely related to the caliber of the distal runoff artery. This suggested that FIH progressed until the vein lumen matched that of the artery. FIH then ceased because the flow had become less turbulent and, therefore, less damaging to the endothelial cells.[39,40] This has led to speculation that some autoregulatory mechanism related to endothelial cell function acts as a transducing element,[41] which may determine whether or not FIH progresses to the point of obstructing the lumen.

Atherosclerosis

Atherosclerotic changes can occur in VGs as early as 3 to 6 months postoperatively,[42,43] and by 36 months, 30% of VGs contain atherosclerosis as a histopathological finding.[44] Six years after bypass surgery, angiography reveals significant changes of atherosclerosis in 14% of patent grafts, and occlusion rates increase to 4.5% a year as compared to 2–4% for the first 5 years after grafting.[10] By 10 years, nearly 50% of grafts that were patent at 5 years are occluded, and the incidence of atherosclerosis demonstrated by angiography in the remaining patent grafts rises to 44%.

The rapid progression of atherosclerosis in the large percentage of VGs appears to be caused by a combination of physiological and biochemical factors. First, the role of altered vascular hemodynamics within the graft is an important determinant. Atherogenesis, like FIH, seems to be accelerated when flow velocity and sheer stress are reduced or if the flow departs from a laminar, unidirectional pattern.[45,46] Turbulence and eddy currents may also promote plaque formation.[47] By comparison, the IMA maintains the normal flow pattern, which may assist in the prevention of the atherosclerotic development. Second, biochemical changes are taking place in transplanted SVs (Table 3), of which the role of lipid metabolism may be the most determinant. Experimentally, autogenous VGs in animals fed a hypercholesterolemic diet were especially susceptible to atheromatous changes.[48] Also, venous tissue, when compared to arterial tissue under hyperlipidemic conditions, had a greater affinity to take up lipids.[19] There is additional evidence that lipid accumulation (measured by the uptake of low density lipoprotein (LDL) 3) is significantly present and that VGs manifest an increased tendency to synthesize complex lipids. Apoproteins and probably lipoproteins also accumulate in human VGs of long duration.[49] Of these, the plasma apolipoprotein (apo) B level may correlate more with the lipid buildup than does the LDL or total serum cholesterol level. Just as there is strong specific experimental evidence for lipid accumulation in VGs, well-documented clinical evidence exists to show that an elevated triglyceride level is strongly associated with the need for repeat bypass surgery.[50] Atherosclerotic development in VGs is also more prevalent in patients with hypercholesterolemia.[51]

Other biochemical activity may set up the VG to develop atherosclerosis. Degranulation of platelets with the release of thromboxane A2 and activation of neutrophils caused by a cardiopulmonary bypass may cause extensive endothelial detachment and damage.[52] This could cause the VG wall to become increasingly susceptible to very early lipid intrusion. Immunoglobulins have also been identified in SVs with diffuse atherosclerosis.[53] These substances could form immune complexes with lipoproteins within the SV wall, stimulating phagocytosis by monocytes and macrophages to form foam cells and foreign body giant cells. C3-binding proteins, too, have been found in plaques. This finding suggests that complement activation may play a role in atherogenesis.[54] These complement reactions may provide yet another mechanism by which monocytes can be attracted to regions of lipid accumulation, particularly in hypercholesterolemic conditions.[55] These and no doubt other yet unidentified biochemical (primarily lipid) interactions contribute to the progression of SV atherogenesis and occlusion.

Even with a superficial understanding of the biological and biochemical forces acting on the VG, a few rational interventions can be developed to improve both short- and long-term graft patency. The use of a meticulous surgical technique during the harvest of the vein, the prevention of overdistribution, and attempts to reduce ischemic injury will help lessen graft injury.[56] Antiplatelet drugs used in the early postgraft period may improve both the short- and long-term patency rates.[28] Lipid modification may also have merit and enhance graft longevity.[57] Finally, whenever possible, the segments of vein being used should be void of valves, areas of dilatation, and severe wall thickening. They should also match closely the size of the arterial bed to be bypassed. This enables maximum benefit to be obtained from the SV as a conduit for coronary revascularization and enhances the likelihood of further improvement with patency rates. In conclusion, with increased usage of the IMA and other arterial conduits and methods of surgical coronary revascularization discussed in this book, surgeons will need to decide case by case whether the SV graft is a standard conduit or an alternative.

References

1. Sabiston DC Jr. Direct surgical management of congenital and acquired lesions of the coronary artery. Prog Cardiovasc Dis 1963; 6:299–316.
2. Garrett HE, Dennis EW, DeBakey ME. Aortocoronary bypass with saphenous vein graft: seven year follow-up. JAMA 1973; 223:792–794.

3. Favaloro R. Saphenous vein autograft replacement of severe segmental coronary artery occlusion. Ann Thorac Surg 1968; 5:335–339.

4. Johnson WD, Flemma RJ, Lepley D Jr. Extended treatment of severe coronary artery disease. Ann Surg 1969; 170:460–470.

5. Bartley TD, Bigelow JC, Page US. Aortocoronary bypass grafting with multiple sequential anastomosis to a single vein. Arch Surg 1972; 105:915–917.

6. Flemma RJ, Singh HM, Tector AJ, Lepley D Jr, et al. Comparative hemodynamics properties of vein and mammary artery in coronary bypass operation. Ann Thorac Surg 1975; 20:619–635.

7. Wakabayaski A, Beron E, Lou MA, Mino JY, et al. Physiological basis for the systemic to coronary artery bypass graft. Arch Surg 1970; 100:17–19.

8. Grondin CM, Lesperance J, Dourassa MG, Pasternac A, et al. Serial angiographic evaluation in 60 consecutive patients with aortocoronary artery vein grafts 2 weeks, 1 year and 3 years after operation. J Thorac Cardiovasc Surg 1974; 67:1–6.

9. Fitzgibbon GM, Leach AJ, Leon WJ, Burton JR, et al. Coronary bypass graft fate: angiographic study of 1,179 vein grafts early, one year, and five years after operation. J Thorac Cardiovasc Surg 1986; 91:773–778.

10. Grondin CM, Lesperance J, Solymoss BC, Vouche P, et al. Atherosclerotic changes in coronary grafts six years after operation. J Thorac Cardiovasc Surg 1979; 77:24–31.

11. Grondin CM, Campeau L, Lesperance J, Enjalbert M, et al. Comparison of late changes in internal mammary artery and saphenous vein grafts in two consecutive series of patients 10 years after operation. Circulation 1984; 70(suppl.I):I-208–I-212.

12. Campeau L, Enjalbert M, Bourassa MG, Lesperance J. Improvement of angina and survival 1 to 12 years after aortocoronary bypass surgery: correlations with changes in grafts and in the native coronary circulation. J Heart Transplant 1984; 220–223.

13. Stanley JC, Ernst CB, Fry WJ. Fate of aortorenal vein grafts: characteristics of late graft expansion, aneurysmal dilatation, and stenosis. Surgery 1973; 74:931–944.

14. Milroy CM, Scott JA, Beard JD, et al. Histological appearances of the long saphenous vein. J Pathol 1984; 159:311–316.

15. Cox JL, Chiasson DA, Gotlieb AI. Stranger in a strange land: the pathogenesis of saphenous vein graft stenosis with emphasis on structural and functional differences between veins and arteries. Prog Cardiovasc Dis 1991; 34:45–68.

16. Simionescu M, Simionescu N, Palade GE. Sequential differentiation of cell junctions in the vascular endothelium: arteries and veins. J Cell Biol 1976; 68:705–723.

17. Palumbo JD, Blackburn GL, Forse RM. Collective review: endothelial cell factors and response to injury. Surg Gynecol Obstet 1991; 173:505–518.

18. Wesly RLR, Valishnav RN, Fuchs JCA, et al. Static linear and nonlinear elastic properties of normal and arterialized venous tissue in dog and man. Circ Res 1975; 37:509–520.

19. Larson RM, Hagen PO, Oldham HN Jr, et al. Lipid biosynthesis in arteries, veins, and venous grafts. Circulation 1974; 50:III-139.

20. Henderson VJ, Mitchell RS, Cohen RG, et al. Recovery of prostacyclin production in venoarterial autografts and allografts. Surg Forum 1984; 35:421–422.
21. Skidegel RA, Printz MP. PGI2 production by rat blood vessels: diminished prostacylin formation in veins compared to arteries. Prostaglandins 1989; 16:1–16.
22. Reichle FA, Stewart GJ, Essa N. A transmission and scanning electron microscopic study of luminal surfaces in dacron and autogenous vein bypasses in man and dog. Surgery 1975; 74:945–960.
23. Fuster V, Dewanjee MK, Kaye MP, et al. Noninvasive radioisotopic technique for detection of platelet deposition in coronary artery bypass grafts in dogs and its reduction with platelet inhibitors. Circulation 1979; 60:1508–1512.
24. Quist WC, Haudenschild CC, LoGerfo FW. Qualitative microscopy of implanted vein grafts. J Thorac Cardiovasc Surg 1992; 103:671–676.
25. Bonchek LF. Prevention of endothelial damage during preparation of saphenous vein for bypass grafting. J Thorac Cardiovasc Surg 1980; 79:911–915.
26. Barner HB. Endothelial preservation in human saphenous veins harvested for coronary grafting. J Thorac Cardiovasc Surg 1990; 100:148–149.
27. Solberg S, Larsen T, Jorgensen L, et al. Cold induced endothelial cell detachment in human saphenous vein grafts. J Cardiovasc Surg 1987; 28:571–575.
28. Bush HL, McCabe ME, Nabseth DC. Functional injury of vein graft endothelium: role of hypothermia and distention. Arch Surg 1984; 119:770–774.
29. Chesebro JM, Clements IP, Fuster V, et al. A platelet inhibitor drug trial in coronary artery bypass operations. Benefit of perioperative dipyridamole and aspirin therapy on early postoperative vein graft patency. N Engl J Med 1982; 307:73–78.
30. Chesebro JM, Fuster V. Platelet-inhibitor drugs before and after coronary artery bypass surgery and coronary angioplasty: the basis of their use, date from animal studies, clinical trial data, and current recommendations. Cardiology 1986; 73:292–305.
31. De Laria GA, Hunter JA, Goldin MD, Serry C, et al. Leg wound complications associated with coronary revascularization. J Thorac Cardiovasc Surg 1981; 81:403–407.
32. Oschner JL, Mills HL. Coronary Artery Surgery. Malvern, Pa.:Lea & Febiger, 1978:161.
33. Virmani R, Atkinson JB, Forman MB. Aortocoronary saphenous vein bypass grafts. Cardiovasc Clin 1988; 18:41–59.
34. Dobrin PB, Littsoy FN, Endian ED. Mechanical factors predisposing to intimal hyperplasia and medial thickening in autogenous vein grafts. Surgery 1989; 105:393–400.
35. Grondin CM, Lepage G, Castonguay Y, et al. Aorto-coronary venous bypass grafts: intimal blood flow through the graft and early post-operative patency. Circulation 1970(suppl. 3); 52:III-106 (abstract).
36. Bernhard VM. Intraoperative monitoring of femorotibial bypass grafts. Surg Clin North Am 1974; 54:77–84.

37. Smith SH, Green JC. Morphology of saphenous vein-coronary artery bypass grafts. Arch Pathol Lab Med 1983; 107:13–18.
38. Brody WR, Kosek JC, Angell WW. Changes in vein grafts following aortocoronary bypass induced by pressure and ischemia. J Thorac Cardiovasc Surg 1972; 64:846–854.
39. Rittgers SE, Karayannacos PE, Guy JF, et al. Velocity distribution and intimal proliferation in autologous vein grafts in dogs. Circ Res 1978; 42:792–801.
40. Zwolak RM, Adams MC, Clowes AW. Kinetics of vein graft hyperplasia: association with tangential stress. J Vasc Surg 1987; 5:126–136.
41. Barboriah JJ, Pintar K. Korns ME. Atherosclerosis in aortocoronary vein grafts. Lancet 1974; 2:621–624.
42. Grondin GM. Graft disease in patients with coronary bypass grafting. Why does it start? Where do we stop? J Thorac Cardiovasc Surg 1986; 92:323–329.
43. Caro CG, Fitzgerald JM, Schroter RC. Atheroma and arterial wall shear: observation, correlation and proposal of a shear dependent mass transfer mechanism for atherogenesis. Proc R Soc Lond [Biol] 1971; 177:109–159.
44. Fuchs JCA, Mitchner JS, Hagen PO. Postoperative changes in autologous vein grafts. Ann Surg 1978; 188:1–15.
45. Mustard JF, Packham MA, Kinlough-Rathbone RL. Platelets, blood flow, and the vessel wall. Circulation 1990(suppl. 1); 81:I24–I27.
46. Fox JA, Hugh AE. Localization of atheroma: a theory based on boundary layer separation. Br Heart J 1966; 28:388–399.
47. Stein PO, Sabbah HN. Measured turbulence and its effect on thrombus formation. Circ Res 1974; 35:608–614.
48. Scott HW, Morgan CV, Bolasny BL, et al. Experimental atherogenesis in autogenous venous grafts. Arch Surg 1970; 101:677–681.
49. Cushing GL, Ganbaty JW, Nava ML, et al. Quantitation and localization of apolipoproteins [a] and B in coronary artery bypass vein grafts resected at reoperation. Arteriosclerosis 1989; 9:593–603.
50. Fox MH, Grachow HW, Barboriah JJ, et al. Risk factors among patients undergoing repeat aortocoronary bypass procedures. J Thorac Cardiovasc Surg 1987; 93:56–61.
51. Bulkley BH, Hutchings GM. Accelerated "atherosclerosis": Amorphologic study of 97 saphenous vein coronary artery bypass grafts. Circulation 1977: 55:163–169.
52. Colman RW. Platelet and neutrophil activation in cardiopulmonary bypass. Ann Thorac Surg 1990; 49:32–34.
53. Ratliff NB, Myles JL. Rapidly progressive atherosclerosis in aortocoronary saphenous vein graft. Possible immune-mediated disease. Arch Pathol Lab Med 1989; 113:772–776.
54. Hardin NJ, Minich CR, Murphy GE. Experimental induction of atheroarteriosclerosis by the synergy of allergic injury to arteries and lipid-rich diet. III: The role of earlier acquired fibromuscular thickening in the pathogenesis of later developing atherosclerosis. Am J Pathol 1973; 73:301–327.
55. Seifert PS, Hugo F, Hanson GK, et al. Prelesional complement activation in experimental atherosclerosis: transluminal C5b-9 complement deposi-

tion coincides with cholesterol accumulation in the aortic intima of hypercholesterolemic rabbits. Lab Invest 1989; 60:747–754.

56. Grondin CM, Lepage G, Castonguay YR, et al. Aortocoronary vein graft: technical modifications that improve short and long-term results. Can J Surg 1973; 16:261–267.

57. Blankenhorn DH, Nessim SA, Johnson RL, et al. Beneficial effects of combined colestipol-niacin therapy on coronary atherosclerosis and coronary venous bypass grafts. JAMA 1987; 257:3233–3240.

Part II
Alternative Venous Bypass Conduits

Chapter 3

The Lesser Saphenous Vein

Ronald K. Grooters and Hiroshi Nishida

The lesser (short) saphenous vein (SV) is not a first choice as a conduit for coronary revascularization, but if other conduits are unavailable, inadequate, or unsuitable, this vein is certainly recommended. The vein is frequently spared from severe varicosities and seems to have fewer sclerotic changes than does the greater SV. It has also been observed that the vein is frequently spared from a stripping procedure. Most important, what makes this vein a very satisfactory alternative venous conduit is that, in a limited study, its patency rates seem comparable to the greater SV.[1]

Anatomy

The lesser SV generally originates posterior to the lateral malleolus as it lies in the subcutaneous tissue and courses cephalad between the heads of the gastrocnemius muscle. It then enters the popliteal fossa and connects to the popliteal vein. One must keep in mind that the sural nerve parallels the vein in the lower half of the calf and that the medial sural cutaneous nerve is in proximity to the vein at the upper part of the calf (Fig. 1). Care should be taken not to damage these structures, which can also be used as important landmarks during the dissection.

From Grooters RK and Nishida H: (editors): *Alternative Bypass Conduits and Methods for Surgical Coronary Revascularization.* © Futura Publishing Co., Inc., Armonk, NY, 1994.

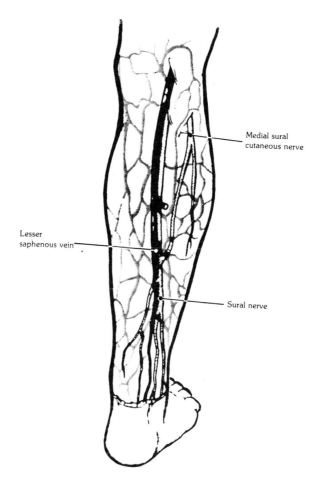

Medial sural
cutaneous nerve

Lesser
saphenous vein

Sural nerve

Fig. 1. The lesser SV as depicted in the right leg viewed posteriorly. Note the close proximity of the sural nerve and the medial cutaneous sural nerve (from Raess DH, et al.[4]).

Removal Techniques

The removal (harvest) of the lesser SV is relatively easy and is accomplished by several methods. First, the patient can be placed in the prone position. This direct approach is extremely easy but two problems must be addressed.

(1) The patient needs to be hemodynamically stable and be kept stable. If the patient's hemodynamics are questionable, then before

starting the harvest the patient should be immediately placed in the supine position.

(2) There may be a prolonged ischemic time before the vein can be used. This delay would potentially cause damage to the endothelial cells. To prevent ischemia, heparinized blood should be available both to test and store the vein until the patient can be turned to the supine position and the bypass procedure commenced.

More frequently, the vein is dissected with the patient in the supine position. This can be accomplished by flexing the hip 45° and the knees at 90° and then internally rotating the hip. This position exposes the lateral aspect of the calf.

The surgeon then is positioned on the patient's ipsilateral side to harvest vein from the lower half of the calf. The popliteal fossa is more difficult to expose with this position. As the upper half of the calf is approached, the surgeon needs to work from the patient's contralateral side as an assistant provides flexion of the hip and knees and external rotation of the hip (Fig 2). Using this approach, addi-

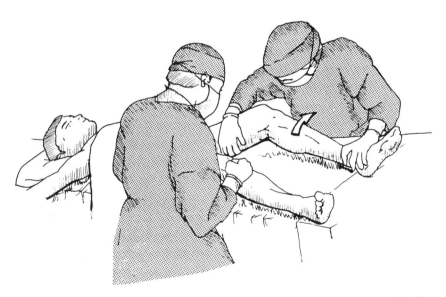

Fig. 2. Operative approach to the lesser SV. An assistant (on patient's left) provides exposure by slightly flexing the patient's hip and knee. The posterior calf is then gently rotated into view. The initial incision is made over the distal extent of the gastrocnemius between the two heads. The surgeon is standing on the patient's right (from Raess DH, et al.[4]).

tional length of the vein can easily be exposed and removed from the popliteal fossa.

Clinical Results

In spite of its preferable aspects, there are no extensive studies reviewing the lesser SV vein as a coronary bypass conduit. In 1975, success was reported using the lesser SV in three patients.[2] It was suggested that its suitability can be demonstrated preoperatively by the application of a venous tourniquet or by venography. Five months after the operations, one of these patients had a coronary angiography that revealed all four grafts to be patent. Salerno and Charrette[3] reported three successful coronary bypass operations using the lesser SV; another study in 1986[4] described six patients with good symptomatic relief, but postoperative catheterizations were not part of either report. The most recent report by Grimball et al.[5] described success using the vein as a conduit for both coronary bypass as well as femoral-popliteal bypass. We have added two additional patients to the eight patients we have previously reported.[6] All ten patients had satisfactory treadmill tests done 8 weeks postoperatively, but no long-term results are available. All wounds healed nicely without significant limb edema.

In conclusion, this vein is of optimal length (25–30 cm) and diameter (usually 2.5–3.5 mm) and of an assumed structure closely related to the greater SV. Although its long-term patency rate is still unknown, the lesser SV could be presumed to be close to that of the great vein.

References

1. Weaver FA, Barlow CR, Edwards WH, et al. The lesser saphenous vein: autogenous tissue for lower extremity revascularization. J Vasc Surg 1987; 5:687.
2. Crosby IK, Carver JM. The lesser saphenous vein. Ann Thorac Surg 1975; 20:703–705.
3. Salerno TA, Charrette EJP. The short saphenous vein: an alternative to the long saphenous vein for aortocoronary bypass. Ann Thorac Surg 1978; 25:457–458.
4. Raess DH, Mahomed Y, Brown JW, et al. Lesser saphenous vein as an alternative conduit of choice in coronary bypass operations. Ann Thorac Surg 1986; 41:334–336.
5. Grimball A, Bradham RR, Lochlair PR Jr. Utility of lesser saphenous vein as a substitute conduit. JSC Med Assoc 1989; 85:226–227.
6. Nishida H, Grooters RK, Soltanzadeh H, Thieman KC, et al. Clinical alternative bypass conduits and methods for surgical coronary revascularization. Surg Gynecol Obstet 1991; 172:161–174.

Chapter 4

The Arm Vein

Ronald K. Grooters and Hiroshi Nishida

In 1969, Kakkar[1] was the first to report the use of the arm vein to graft an artery. Cephalic veins were used as femoropopliteal bypass grafts in 8 patients, and all were found to be patent 4–12 months postoperatively. Schulman and Badhay[2] used 68 arm veins exclusively in the femoropopliteal position and reported in 1982 that most of the conduits rapidly developed intimal hyperplasia and occluded. The few that were still patent elongated and became aneurysmal. Stoney et al.[3] found the long-term patency of the arm vein in the coronary-bypass position to be only 57% at 2 years. The best results were reported by Jarvinen and associates[4] in 1984 (Table 1). In arm vein grafts for 15 patients, 87.1% of the anastomoses were patent in the follow-up period of 1 year or more.

In addition to these variable and questionable patency rates, surgeons have found the arm vein to be thin, delicate, and very difficult to dissect. Distention and intravenous injections easily traumatize and impair the functioning of the vein. These problems raise the question of whether the arm vein should be used and when, particularly since it has been shown that cumulative patency rates of the arm vein show increased progressive failure when compared to the internal mammary artery (IMA) and saphenous vein (SV) (Fig.1).[3]

Indications

There are no definitive indications for use of the arm vein as a conduit in the coronary position, but some conditions seem logical to consider before using it.

From Grooters RK and Nishida H: (editors): *Alternative Bypass Conduits and Methods for Surgical Coronary Revascularization.* © Futura Publishing Co., Inc., Armonk, NY, 1994.

Table 1

Angiographic Patency of Arm Veins in Coronary Bypass Positions

Author	Year	Number of Patients Bypassed	Number of Anastomoses	Early: Number & Percentage	Late: Number & Percentage
Parsonnet*[10]	1976	1	1	1/1 100%*	—
Seifert[11]	1982	21	44	23/25 65.7%	—
Stoney[3]	1984	59	—	32/56 57.1%	—
Jarvinen[4]	1984	15	34	—	27/31 87.1%
Prieto[5]	1984	13	35	9/10 90%	5/8 62.5%
Norman[7]	1991	55	4	—	3/4 75%
Mehta**[6]	1991	1	2	—	2/2 100%

*graft wrapped with polypropylene mesh; **grafts arterialized with fistulization 2 weeks prior to surgery—one graft patent at 7 years and one graft patent at 11 years

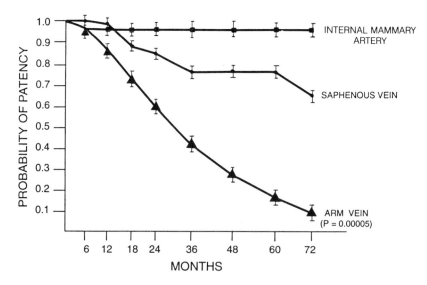

Fig. 1. Cumulative patency rates of arm vein, internal mammary, and saphenous vein grafts. The arm vein grafts show progressive failure with each year (from Stoney WS, et al.[3]).

(1) The IMAs and SVs should be absent, unavailable, or inadequate.

(2) The nonroutine arterial conduits such as the right gastroepiploic artery (RGEA), the inferior epigastric artery (IEA), and even the radial artery (RA) as well as the lesser SV should be considered first, if present.

(3) Percutaneous transluminal coronary angioplasty (PTCA) must be given consideration, particularly if the coronary stenosis looks suitable and safe to dilate. This seems reasonable since the one-year patency of arm veins is only 62%,[5] not much better than PTCA at 1 year.

(4) Surgeons need to consider the clinical stability of the patient to determine if a few weeks are available before surgery to "arterialize" the arm vein conduits. The case report by Mehta and associates[6] shows that a long-term patency graft patency from 7 to 11 years with arterialized arm veins may make this option attractive.

Pathophysiology of Arm Vein Occlusion

A plausible hypothesis for the high occlusive rate of the arm vein was explained by Norman and associates.[7] They concluded that the upper-extremity blood flow is approximately one-half that of the lower-extremity flow. The arm vein conduits, therefore, teleologically have one half the tensile strength of the SV system when placed in the aortocoronary position. Arterial hemodynamic forces, along with the degradation of wall elastin, then cause the vein to elongate, become tortuous, and aneurysmal soon after the implantation.[8] Boundary layer flow phenomena are then disrupted as turbulence occurs, and the tendency to thrombose rapidly increases. To overcome the problem, Beals[9] created an arteriovenous fistula to toughen, gradually dilate, and thicken the vein. He reported a series of 40 side-to-side anastomoses between the radial artery and the cephalic vein. These veins gradually became "arterialized" and increase from 2–4 mm in diameter to 4–6 mm within a few weeks. Wall thickness increased, and the veins were much more durable. Mehta and associates[6] successfully used an end-to-side anastomosis of the cephalic vein to the RA. Two weeks later, the arm vein was used as a coronary bypass graft to the right coronary artery and the obtuse marginal coronary artery. These arterialization methods look promising and may allow the vein to accommodate and resist the new pathophysiological environment of the aortocoronary artery position. Parsonnet et al.[10] took a different approach by using a sleeve of polypropylene mesh. He demonstrated angiographically that aneurysmal dilatation could be successfully prevented.

Clinical Results in the Coronary Position

The high failure rate both short term (1 year) and long term for the arm vein is a distressing and unacceptable problem, especially when compared to the IMA and the SV (Fig. 1). The angiographic patency rates are also reported differently for each author (Table 1) but do share a consistent failure rate. Stoney et al.[3] reported only a 57% patency rate studied by recatheterization at a mean 25 months following bypass surgery. Prieto[5] was not much better with a 62% patency rate at 1 year (5 of 8 arm veins patent), but significant abnormalities were found in 2 of the patent grafts. In 1984, Jarvinen et al.[4] reported the best results with an 87.1% patency rate at 1.4 years. Arm veins in three of his patients developed aneurysmal dilatation. Seifert et al.[11] reported a patency rate for arm veins of 65.7% but only at 8 months after surgery. Norman[7] also experienced suboptimal results with 37 of 55 patients alive from 1 to 10 years, but 9 of the 37 patients had recurrent angina. Of the 28 patients without symptoms 2 to 4 years postoperatively, only 4 patients were studied angiographically. Three of the arm veins were patent. The best long-term patency result to date is reported by Mehta and associates,[6] but it is only a case report. They used an "arterialized" arm vein for two grafts, one of which was patent angiographically up to 7 years and the second at 11 years postoperatively.

Conclusion

For the most part, cephalic and basilic arm veins have disappointing patency rates. They should be used only if other arterial conduits and the lesser SV are not feasible or present. If time permits, the surgeon may want to consider "arterializing" the vein using a radial artery-vein fistula. Additionally, angiography should be used annually for patients in whom arm veins are used as coronary conduits, particularly if the arm veins bypass vessels that supply large segments of myocardium. Stoney et al.[3] has suggested this frequent follow-up so that if stenosis develops, failure of the graft can be avoided by early detection, and the graft may be treated with a transluminal dilatation.

References

1. Kakkar VV. The cephalic vein as a peripheral vascular graft. Surg Gynecol Obstet 1969; 128:551–556.
2. Schulman ML, Badhey MR. Late results and angiographic evaluation of arm veins as long bypass grafts. Surgery 1982; 92:1032–1041.
3. Stoney WS, Alford WC Jr, Burrus GR, Glassford DM, et al. The fate of arm veins used for aortocoronary bypass grafts. J Thorac Cardiovasc Surg 1984; 84:522–526.
4. Jarvinen A, Harjula A, Mattila S, Volle M, et al. Experience with arm veins as aortocoronary bypass grafts. J Cardiovasc Surg 1984; 25:344–347.
5. Prieto I, Basile F, Abdulnom E. Upper extremity vein graft for aortocoronary bypass. Ann Thorac Surg 1984; 36:218–221.
6. Mehta S, Levine S, Marjolis JR, Martin JC, et al. Long-term patency of arterialized cephalic veins used as a conduit for coronary artery bypass grafting. Cathet Cardiovasc Diagn 1991; 23:208–210.
7. Norman JC, Lansing AM, Yared SF. Cephalic/basilic veins for aortocoronary bypass: review, report and analyze. J Ky Med Assoc 1991; 89:67–70.
8. Dobrin PB, Schwarez TH, Baker SH. Mechanisms of arterial and aneurysmal tortuosity. Surgery 1988; 104:568–571.
9. Beals RL. Surgically created arteriovenous fistula to augment the cephalic vein: use as an arterial bypass graft. N Engl J Med 1971; 285:29–30.
10. Parsonnet V, Alpert J, Brief DK. Autogenous polypropylene supported collagen tubes for long-term arterial replacement. Surgery 1971; 70:935.
11. Seifert D, Bircks W, Jehle BJ, et al. Aortocoronary bypass grafts using cephalic veins. Thorac Cardiovasc Surg 1982; 30:15–16.

Chapter 5

The Homologous Veins

Ronald K. Grooters and Hiroshi Nishida

It appears that use of homologous venous conduits in the aorto-coronary position has been abandoned. The poor patency rates reported by all the authors (Table 1) definitely supports this condemnation. In the past, these veins looked like possibilities, particularly when only the autogenous saphenous vein (SV) was held up as the standard, but now that many other arterial conduits and alternative bypass methods have been formed to provide excellent results, the homologous venous conduit becomes only of historical interest when used in the coronary position.

Fresh Homologous Saphenous Vein

Fresh homologous saphenous veins (SVs) had been previously used for arterial reconstruction as femoral popliteal bypasses by Ochsner et al.[1] in 1971. The occlusion rate was 50% (11 of 22 grafts) in the follow-up period of 3–48 months. The 6 grafts that remained patent 1 year or more were ABO compatible, while all ABO incompatible veins were occluded at 6 months. This work suggested that fresh homologous vein grafts develop a rejection reaction that produced premature fibrosis and occlusion of the grafts within 1 year in most cases.

The only complete report of fresh homologous SVs used in the coronary position was presented by Bical and associates[2] in 1980. Seven fresh grafts were harvested from living, nonrelated donors and stored in 4°C saline solution containing penicillin. The conduits were then used as aortocoronary bypasses within 24 hours in seven pa-

From Grooters RK and Nishida H: (editors): *Alternative Bypass Conduits and Methods for Surgical Coronary Revascularization.* © Futura Publishing Co., Inc., Armonk, NY, 1994.

Table 1
Homologous Vein Graft Patency

Author	Year	Type of Preservation	Number of Patients	Number of Anastomoses	Early: Number & Percentage	Late: Number & Percentage
Bical[2]	1980	fresh	4	7	—	2/7 28.5%
Tice[3]	1976	cryo*	13	19	—	6/8 75.0%
Bical[2]	1980	cryo*	20	27	6/7 85.7%	2/10 20.0%
Bhayana[4]	1980	cryo*	7	22	19/22 86.0%	—
Gelbfish	1980	cryo*	28	61	23/31 74.2% 2/13 15.4%	—
Silver[10]	1982	glut**	11	22	6/12 50.0%	—

Early: mean follow-up period of less than 1 year; Late: mean follow-up of more than 1 year; * cryo: cyropreserved homologous vein; ** glut: glutaraldehyde umbilical vein tients. Angiography in the period up to 44 months after surgery found five of the seven fresh veins to be occluded.

Cryopreserved Homologous Saphenous Vein

In 1976, Tice and colleagues[3] used the cryopreserved homologous saphenous vein graft in 13 patients. The veins were prepared after harvesting by irrigation with physiological Ringer's lactate solution containing penicillin and streptomycin and then stored at $-50°C$. There were no operative deaths.

At 1 year after surgery, 30.7% (4 of 13) of the patients had died. Unfortunately, no autopsies were obtained. Six of the survivors underwent angiography 3 weeks to 42 months after bypass surgery, and 5 of the 8 cryopreserved veins grafts were patent.

Then, in 1980, Bical and associates[2] reported on the use of 20 homologous veins cryopreserved in glycerol at a temperature of $-40°C$. The patency rate of 86% (6 of 7 veins) during the early postoperative period at 3 months or less had decreased to 20% (2 of 10 veins) in the 8 to 68 months after revascularization. Bhayana[4] in a comment to the report by Bical reported the use of homologous veins stored in Plasmanate (Cutter Biologicals, Emeryville, Calif.) containing cephalothin at $-60°C$ in seven patients. There was one operative death. The 6 surviving patients underwent angiography 4–12 months postsurgery and had an early graft patency rate of 86% (19 of 22 grafts). ABO compatibility between the donor and the recipient was maintained in this series. Tice and colleagues[3] believe that cryopreservation produces a nonantigenic vein conduit on the basis of the fact that there is little histological evidence of an immune inflammatory reaction after implantation. Barner[5] and other researchers oppose this view and believe, on the basis of experimental evidence, that frozen vein is as antigenic as fresh homologous vein.

By 1980, Gelbfish et al.[6] had used 61 cryopreserved venous homografts in 28 patients. These veins were flushed with a saline solution containing papaverine (60 mg/dl), lidocaine (80 mg/dl), and heparin (2,000 units). The excess vein was cryopreserved in normal saline solution containing 1,000,000 units of penicillin at $-50°C$. Patency was studied angiographically 8 to 12 days postoperatively in 16 patients. Of the 31 homografts studied, 8 were occluded, 3 were stenotic, and 20 were normal. Six patients underwent late catheterization 6 to 12 months after surgery. Thirteen homografts were studied; 11 were occluded, 1 was severely stenotic, and 1 was mildly stenotic. They concluded that the use of cryopreserved homologous SVs of coronary artery bypass grafting should be avoided if at all possible.

Glutaraldehyde-Tanned Homologous Saphenous Vein

Although the glutaraldehyde-tanned homologous saphenous vein has been used and investigated, we can find no published clinical reports. We can recall using this conduit in two patients approximately 10 years ago and remember that the vein was so stiff and the lumen so nondistensible that we were concerned that the graft would not stay open. One of those patients died of a massive postoperative myocardial infarction 3 days postbypass. The infarction occurred in the myocardial segment supplied by the tanned vein graft. No autopsy was obtained. This incident stopped us from using this type of graft.

Glutaraldehyde-Treated Homologous Umbilical Vein

Previous animal work done by Dardik et al.[7] in 1976 provided excellent objective data for the glutaraldehyde-preserved homologous umbilical vein to be used clinically. This graft did extremely well when used for arteriovenous (AV) fistulas[8] and for peripheral vascular bypasses.[9] In 1980, Silver et al.[10] reported his experience with the human umbilical vein and its pitfalls when used as an aortocoronary conduit.

Only coronary vessels at least 1.5 mm in diameter were selected for his study. Meticulous technique and special attention to details were thought to be essential to achieve a satisfactory result. First, thorough irrigation of the biograft by a knowledgeable nurse was essential to prevent intimal damage. Second, the internal elastic lamina surrounded by the layer of smooth muscle actually represented the intima of the biograft. This internal elastic lamina was known to have very good surface characteristics and blood compatibility but did have a tendency to dissect easily. Silver thus developed a "no-touch" technique to prevent the dissection of the intima when constructing the anastomoses. Third, it was found that the graft was flexible, had good circumferential elasticity, and would distend with arterial pressure. However, it lacked linear elasticity and, thus, the length of the graft was a critical measurement to prevent kinking.

Eleven patients were involved in the study. There was one operative death. The umbilical vein graft was found to be occluded at autopsy. Three to 13 months after bypass surgery, 6 of the 10 survivors had coronary angiography. The patency rate was 50% (6 of 12 biografts). The analysis of the patients' symptoms and angiographic studies suggested that the graft did well for 3 to 4 months, but longer-term occlusive problems occurred. It was concluded that the glutaraldehyde umbilical vein grafts were nonviable grafts with no antigenicity, but the early patency rates were still a major reason for concern.

Conclusion

It appears that all homologous vein grafts in whatever form are possible to use technically, but the poor patency rates keep this graft in the hazardous category. Many other viable venous and arterial grafts along with unique but successful methods of revascularization techniques described throughout this book need to be considered first.

References

1. Ochsner JL, DeCamp PT, Lenard GL. Experience with fresh venous allografts: an arterial substitute. Ann Surg 1971; 173:933–939.
2. Bical O, Bachet J, Laurian C, Camilleri JP, et al. Aortocoronary bypass with homologous saphenous vein: long-term results. Ann Thorac Surg 1980; 30:550–557.
3. Tice DA, Urbino UR, Isom OW, Cunningham JN, et al. Coronary artery bypass with freeze-preserved saphenous vein allografts. J Thorac Cardiovasc Surg 1976; 71:378–380.
4. Bhayana JN. Discussion of Bical et al. (Ref. 2). Ann Thorac Surg 1980; 30:550–557.
5. Barner HB. Discussion of Bical et al. (Ref. 2). Ann Thorac Surg 1980; 30:550–557.
6. Gelbfish J, Jacobowitz IJ, Rose DM, et al. Cryopreserved homologous saphenous vein. Early and late patency in coronary artery bypass surgical procedures. Ann Thorac Surg 1980; 42.70–73.
7. Dardik H, Dardik I. Successful arterial substitution with modified human umbilical vein. Ann Surg 1976; 183:252–258.

8. Rubio PA. Human umbilical vein graft angio-access in chronic hemodialysis: a preliminary report. Dial Transplant 1979; 8:211.
9. Dardik H, Dardik I, Sproyregen S, et al. Patient selection and improved technical aspects in small vessel bypass procedures of the lower extremities. Surgery 1975; 77:249.
10. Silver GM, Katske GE, Stutzman FL, et al. Umbilical vein for aortocoronary bypass. Angiology 1982; 33:450–453.

Part III
Alternative Arterial Bypass Conduits

Chapter 6

The Right Gastroepiploic Artery Graft

Hisayoshi Suma

The right gastroepiploic artery (RGEA) was used for indirect myocardial revascularization by Bailey,[1] Vineberg,[2] and their colleagues in the 1960s, and Sterling Edwards utilized the RGEA for coronary artery bypass grafting in the early 1970s,[3] though there is no exact documentation. One and one-half decades later, the RGEA was revived as a new arterial conduit following general recognition of the superiority of the internal thoracic artery (ITA) over the saphenous vein (SV) graft in coronary artery bypass grafting.

Anatomy

The RGEA is the largest terminal branch of the gastroduodenal artery, the other branch being the superior pancreaticoduodenal artery (Fig. 1). The gastroduodenal artery arises from the common hepatic artery in 75% of cases, and it may also branch away from the right or left hepatic artery, the accessory left hepatic artery, or the celiac trunk. In a rare case in which the gastroduodenal artery is absent, the RGEA arises from the superior mesenteric artery (Fig. 2). The RGEA may run through an arcade formed by the gastroduodenal artery and the superior mesenteric artery.

The RGEA, which arises from the gastroduodenal branch, runs between the posterior surface of the proximal region of the duodenum and the anterior surface of the pancreas head, along the lower margin of the pylorus, and then along the greater curvature of the

From Grooters RK and Nishida H: (editors): *Alternative Bypass Conduits and Methods for Surgical Coronary Revascularization.* © Futura Publishing Co., Inc., Armonk, NY, 1994.

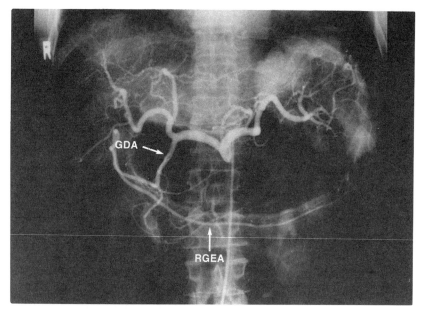

Fig. 1. Celiac angiogram. GDA : gastroduodenal artery; RGEA: right gastro-epiploic artery.

stomach, together with the right gastroepiploic vein toward the left between two layers of the gastrocolic omentum.

Hannoun et al.[4] have reported that the RGEA reached two thirds, one half, and one third of the greater curvature in 58%, 36%, and 6% of cases, respectively, and Suma et al.[5] have reported this to be so in 34%, 61%, and 5% of cases, respectively. Thus, in many cases, the RGEA reaches more than half of the greater curvature of the stomach. The diameter of the RGEA is 3 mm or more at its origin and is 1.5–2 mm in the middle of the greater curvature.[3,6]

The mode of termination of the RGEA is variable. According to a report by Yamato et al.,[7] the RGEA forms a continuous arcade with the left gastroepiploic artery (LGEA) in 35% of cases, forms plexiform anastomoses with the LGEA in 15% of cases, has no communication with the LGEA in 45% of cases, and forms indirect anastomoses through the epiploic artery in 5% of cases.

Surgical Procedure

A midsternal incision is extended to the midpoint between the xiphoid process and the umbilicus. The sternum is incised, the ITA is

GEA via SMA

KI 54M

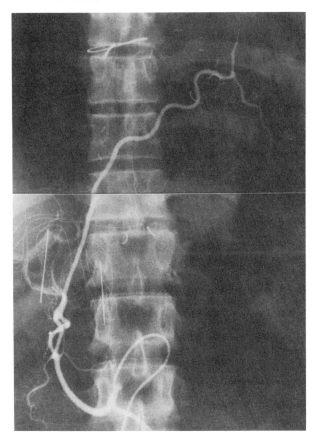

Fig. 2. RGEA arising from the superior mesenteric artery.

taken down, and the peritoneum is opened. The stomach is emptied by nasogastric suction so that surgical manipulation is easier to perform. First, an evaluation of the RGEA by palpation should be performed. The RGEA is liable to become spastic by mechanical stimulation, and after manipulation it is often difficult to estimate its correct size and length. Therefore, it is important that the RGEA be initially handled gently along the greater curvature of the stomach to estimate its thickness, length, and pulse strength.

After inspection of the RGEA, the stomach and the major omentum are laid out, and the RGEA is detached as a pedicle along with the surrounding tissues from the greater curvature. Branches of the RGEA running toward the omentum are then divided and ligated. The branches on the omental side are usually small, and they are easy to divide by electric cautery or the LDS stapler (United States Surgical Corporation, Norwalk, Conn.) Branches running from the RGEA to the stomach should be ligated firmly with silk before they are divided because they are thick and short. If hemostasis at this site is incomplete, hematoma will develop in the RGEA pedicle, making it difficult to stop hemorrhage.

Detachment of the RGEA at the proximal site should be limited to the lower margin of the pylorus, and it is not necessary to extend it to the posterior region of the duodenum. The length of the distal site required for the pedicle varies according to the target coronary artery. Usually, the RGEA is taken down to one half to two thirds of the greater curvature (Figs. 3 and 4). In general, the length of the RGEA to be freed should be as long as possible on the basis of the first estimation of its length and thickness. If the pedicle is too short, serious problems may occur, but a long pedicle causes no problems. It has been demonstrated that detachment of the RGEA from the stomach causes no ischemia of this organ, and no special care is required.[8]

When harvesting of all grafts is completed, a perfusion cannula is then inserted into the ascending aorta, and a single two-stage cannula is inserted from the right atrium to the inferior vena cava under systemic heparinization.

The RGEA is divided distally, then 3–4 mL of diluted papaverine hydrochloride (40 mg in 10 mL of physiological saline) is injected into the lumen to relieve spasm. As shown in Fig. 5, papaverine is injected without proximal clamping of the graft, and then the distal end is clamped so that the artery is dilated by the pharmacological effect and its own pressure. I believe that this procedure will prevent intimal damage due to excessive hydrostatic pressure. Papaverine should also be injected with great care to avoid intimal damage of the artery, and I always use a 22-gauge Quick Cath (Baxter Healthcare Corp., Deerfield, Ill.).

After clamping the distal end of the RGEA, the pedicle is again checked for bleeding. The distance to the site for anastomosis is measured to determine the correct length of the graft. The surrounding tissue of the RGEA adjacent to the site for anastomosis is ligated, and

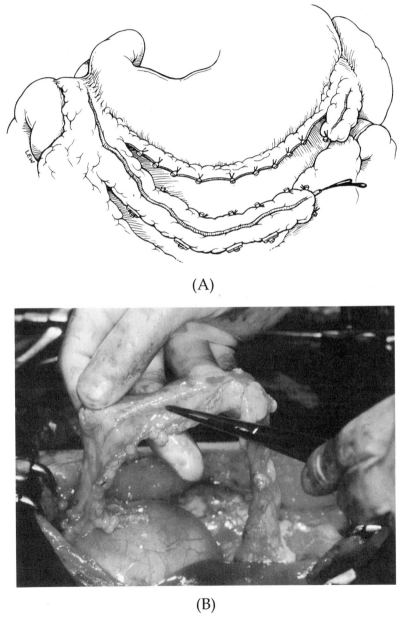

(A)

(B)

Fig. 3. RGEA is taken down along the greater curvature of the stomach as a pedicle containing surrounding tissues.

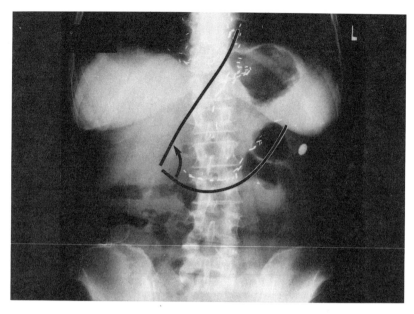

Fig. 4. RGEA is detached from one half to two thirds of the greater curvature of the stomach, which is long enough to reach to major coronary arteries.

2–3 cm of the RGEA is skeletonized. The right gastroepiploic vein running along the RGEA is also ligated. The distal end of the skeletonized RGEA is transsected, cut back to a length of a few millimeters, trimmed for anastomosis, and then checked to ensure free flow.

After injection of papaverine, the free flow rate of the RGEA is usually 80–100 mL/min or more, and this value is similar to that of the ITA in Japanese patients.[9] If the free flow rate is 50 mL/min or less after an intraluminal papaverine injection, the RGEA should not be used for in situ grafting to an important coronary artery. Causes of poor flow include stenosis in the hepatic artery, the gastroduodenal artery, or the RGEA or an anatomical abnormality of RGEA itself.

After trimming the RGEA and upon confirmation of the absence of bleeding from the pedicle along with the presence of good free flow, a hole the size of 1–2 fingers' breadth is made in the diaphragm. The RGEA pedicle is then brought into the pericardial space through this hole. To avoid twisting the pedicle, Mills and Everson[10] have recommended making a mark on the surface of the pedicle with a 2-0 suture. I looked at silk ligations on the branches of the RGEA pedicle to identify any twisting.

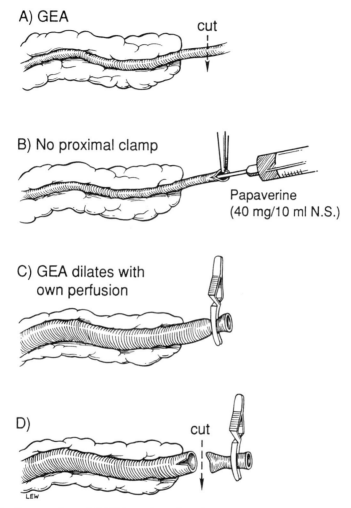

Fig. 5. Preparation of RGEA graft. Diluted papaverine is gently given into the RGEA lumen without proximal clamping. By clamping the distal end thereafter, RGEA dilates by pharmacological effect and its own pressure.

To make a hole in the diaphragm safely and easily, gauze is packed into the space between the diaphragm and the liver, and then the diaphragm is incised from the pericardial space toward the peritoneal cavity by electrocautery (Fig. 6). The size of the hole varies according to the thickness of the pedicle, but it is usually 1–2 fingers' breadth. The location of the hole varies according to the target coro-

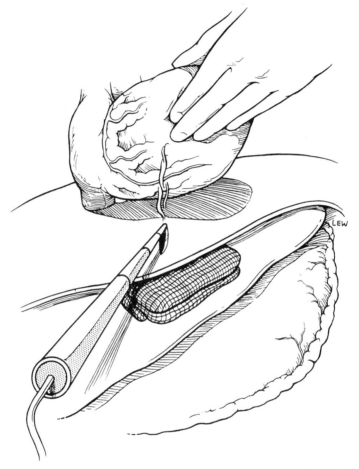

Fig. 6. An appropriate-size hole is made by electrocautery in the diaphragm by packing gauze between the liver and the diaphragm to avoid heat injury to the liver.

nary artery. A hole is made toward the right and anterior for the right coronary artery (RCA) and at the middle posterior site for the circumflex artery (CX). Only a simple incision is made in the anterior diaphragm instead of making a hole for the RGEA grafting of the left anterior descending (LAD).

The RGEA pedicle can be introduced into the pericardial space over the anterior surface of the stomach and the liver (anterior route), or along the posterior surface of these organs (posterior route), or along the posterior surface of the stomach and over the anterior surface of the liver (crossing route).[10] I always use the anterior route because it is easier to check for twisting or bleeding of the pedicle after the completed anastomosis. Although the posterior route might accommodate a shorter graft to the posterior part of the heart, I think that the pedicle is long enough even to bypass the circumflex artery by an anterior route. When the pedicle has been freed almost to the pylorus, there is no risk of stretching the graft even if the stomach is distended by a meal.

After the RGEA pedicle is introduced into the pericardial space through a hole in the diaphragm, the distal end of the pedicle is fixed at the anterior margin of the diaphragm with forceps (Fig. 7). This procedure eliminates the need for an assistant when performing the anastomosis. In this position, a vascular clamp previously applied to the RGEA is released to ensure free flow. If a vigorous free flow is observed, kinking or twisting of the pedicle is considered to be physiologically absent.

When all necessary preparations are made, cardiopulmonary bypass is instituted, and anastomosis of the graft and the coronary artery is performed under moderate hypothermia and cardioplegic arrest. Generally, anastomoses of the free grafts such as the SV or the inferior epigastric artery (IEA) are done first, followed by the ITA and lastly the RGEA.

I perform the anastomosis of the RGEA and the coronary artery using a continuous suture of 7-0 or a 8-0 single polypropylene suture. The RGEA is fixed on the diaphragm, and the continuous suture is applied to the heel of the graft with two to three stitches (Fig. 7). Then, the suture is pulled to approximate the RGEA to the coronary artery, and the continuous suture is continued. After three fourths of the circumference is sutured, a graduated probe is introduced through anastomosis to confirm the patency and then the remaining one fourth is sutured (Fig. 8).

The direction of the anastomosis depends on the site of the anastomosis. When the target is the posterior descending, or low main right coronary artery, the RGEA is anastomosed in antegrade fashion by placing the heel on the proximal end of the anastomosis (Figs. 9, 10). On the other hand, the anastomosis is made in retrograde fashion by placing the heel on the distal aspect of the arteriotomy when the target is the anterior descending artery or, rarely, the high main right coronary artery (Figs. 11,12). For CX the artery, we prefer the

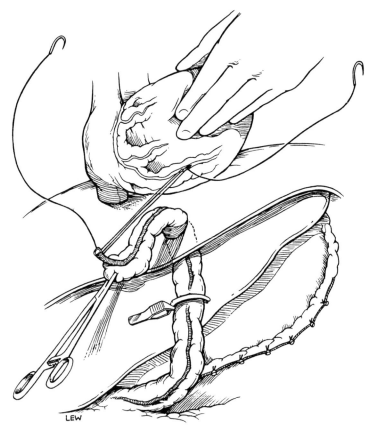

Fig. 7. RGEA pedicle is raised up through the hole in the diaphragm passing the liver and the stomach anteriorly (anterior route), and the end of the pedicle is fixed to the anterior edge of the diaphragm with forceps to facilitate the anastomoses. With a 7-0 or 8-0 polypropylene suture, a few running sutures are placed at the heel of the RGEA and the coronary artery.

antegrade anastomosis (Fig. 13), but this should be decided by the natural relationship between the site of the anastomosis and the course of the graft.

When the anastomosis is completed, the RGEA is unclamped to observe any anastomotic leakage before the aortic crossclamp is released. Then the RGEA pedicle is appropriately fixed to the epicardium near the anastomotic site. At this time, great care should be

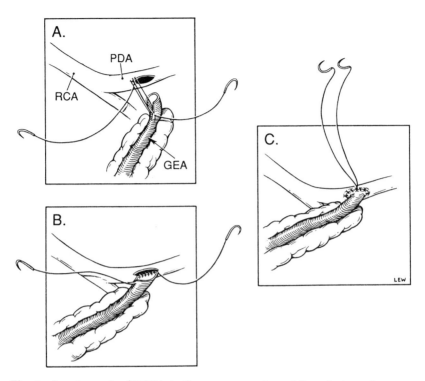

Fig. 8. Anastomosis of RGEA to the coronary artery. After placing a few running sutures at the heel of RGEA (A), the stitch is pulled until the RGEA approximates the coronary artery, then the suture continues up to three fourths of the circumference (B). After probing, the remaining one fourth is closed with the other end of the stitch (C). PDA: posterior descending artery.

taken to prevent kinking or twisting of the skeletonized distal RGEA at the perianastomotic site (Fig. 14).

After the RGEA is correctly fixed to the epicardium, the perfusing RGEA frequently causes a beating of the heart or vigorous ventricular fibrillation. This is good evidence of satisfactory RGEA flow.

With the heart distended to its normal size following release of the aortic crossclamp, the pedicle is observed for correct length and fixation. Excess pedicle, if present, is pulled back into the abdominal cavity. Cardiopulmonary bypass is weaned from the patient, hemostasis is confirmed, and the wound is closed. It is not necessary to introduce a drainage tube into the abdominal cavity.

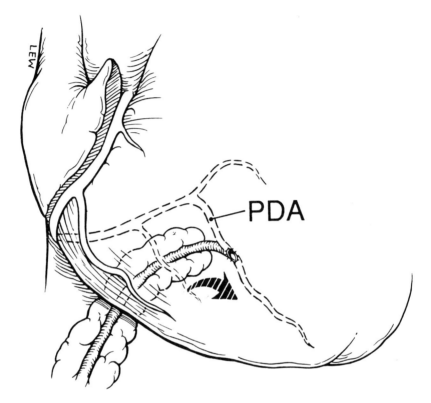

Fig. 9. Antegrade RGEA—coronary artery anastomosis.

Free Right Gastroepiploic Artery (RGEA) Graft

When the RGEA is used as a free graft, preparation of the graft and anastomosis to the coronary artery are performed in the same manner as for in situ grafting. The only difference is that this requires a proximal anastomosis. As shown in Fig. 15, the proximal anastomotic sites for the RGEA include the ascending aorta, a SV graft, an ITA graft, or even the proximal part of the right coronary artery. When the ascending aorta is thickened or has atherosclerotic lesions, direct anastomosis to the ascending aorta should be avoided. If it is necessary to perform the anastomosis on a severely diseased ascending aorta, the anastomosis should be performed using circulatory ar-

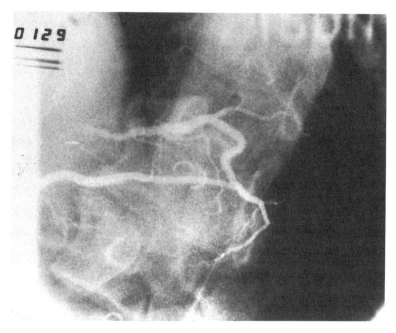

Fig. 10. Angiogram of RGEA—right coronary (posterior descending artery) anastomosis.

rest without clamping the aorta. A soft and thin part of the ascending aorta can easily be detected by palpation under circulatory arrest. The ascending aorta should be incised without the use of a punch-out technique. The anastomosis is carefully performed using a 7-0 polypropylene suture. For similar techniques using the ITA, see Chapters 12, 14, and 15.

Indication for Right Gastroepiploic Artery (RGEA) Grafting

Indications for the RGEA graft have changed with time and experience but may be variable depending on the attitude of the surgeon. In our initial experience, the RGEA was limited to reoperations, a calcified ascending aorta, or the young patient with hyperlipidemia. Now, we utilize the graft more freely as a primary coronary-artery bypass graft because of favorable early and midterm results.

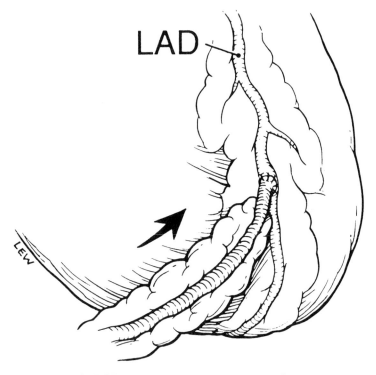

Fig. 11. Retrograde RGEA—coronary artery anastomosis.

While RGEA grafting is questionable in obese or elderly patients or in patients who have had a previous laparotomy or a planned abdominal surgery, the RGEA graft is advantageous for the coronary artery reoperation. The RGEA is usually present and can be harvested before sternal re-entry. The RGEA graft can also be safely and conveniently used for the aortic "no-touch" technique in patients with severely atherosclerotic ascending aorta (see Chapter 23, Fig. 1).[11,12]

Surgical Results

In 1987, Pym,[13] Suma,[5] Carter,[14] and Attum[15] and their coworkers reported RGEA grafting, and now this grafting has been increasingly employed worldwide. Studies reported in English-language papers published up to 1992 account for a sizable number of patients, as listed in Table 1. Carter[14] performed anastomosis of the in situ

GEA–LAD

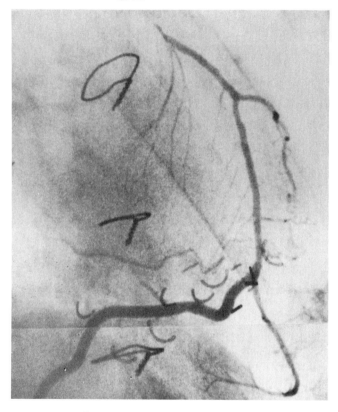

Fig. 12. Angiogram of RGEA—anterior descending artery anastomosis.

RGEA to 35 coronary arteries, including 5 sequential grafts in 30 patients. Target arteries were all posterior descending arteries or the posterolateral branches, and angiography performed early postoperatively revealed that 7 out of 9 RGEAs (78%) were patent. Verkkala et al.[16] used the in situ RGEA to bypass the RCA in 11 patients and found 9 of 11 RGEAs (82%) to be patent. Mills and Everson[3] performed RGEA grafting to a total of 43 coronary arteries, including 2 sequential grafts (5 diagonal, 4 CXs, and 34 RCAs by using 26 in situ grafts and 15 free grafts in 39 patients. They found that all 29 RGEAs studied were patient in the immediate postoperative period. Lytle

GEA–LCX

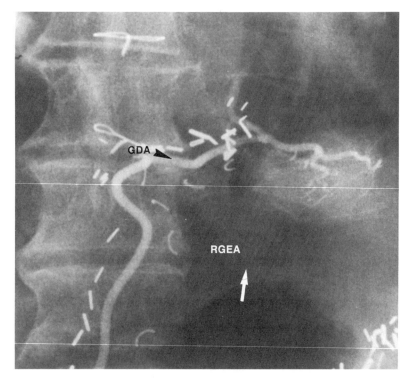

Fig. 13. RGEA–CX artery bypass by antegrade anastomosis.

et al.[17] grafted 6 LAD or diagonal arteries, 8 CX arteries, and 22 RCAs by using 17 in situ RGEA grafts and 19 free grafts in 36 patients. Early angiography revealed that all nine RGEA grafts were patent. In a series of cases reported by Mills and coworkers[3] and Lytle and coworkers,[17] early mortality seemed high, 7.7% and 5.6%, respectively, possibly because the graft was used for the atherosclerotic ascending aorta or a reoperation. The higher mortality was not attributable to the use of the RGEA itself. Beretta et al.[18] performed free grafting in 20 patients using the RGEA on 27 coronary arteries (4 anterior-descending, 1 diagonal, 13 CXs, and 9 RCAs) including 7 sequential grafts. Early angiography revealed that all 20 RGEA grafts

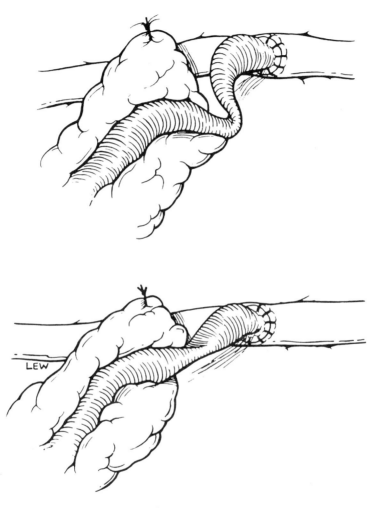

Fig. 14. Kinking and twisting of RGEA due to inappropriate fixation at the perianastomotic site.

were patent. Pym et al.[19] performed bypasses of 5 CX and 52 RCAs using 56 in situ RGEA grafts and 1 free RGEA graft in 57 patients. Imaging revealed 25 of 26 RGEA grafts to be patent. Tanimoto et al.[20] reported using the free RGEA graft divided into two segments to create a Y graft to bypass three coronary arteries. Takeuchi et al.[21] and

PROXIMAL ANASTOMOSIS OF THE FREE GEA GRAFT

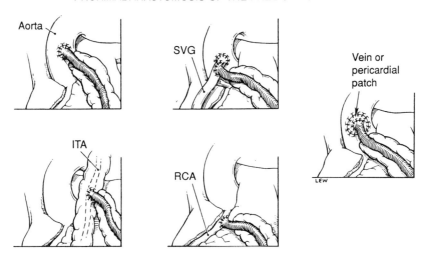

Fig. 15. Sites of proximal anastomosis of the free RGEA graft.

Isomura et al.[22] have both reported successful application of RGEA grafting in pediatric patients with Kawasaki disease.

I have used the RGEA in 223 patients from March 1986 to April 1992. This number was 30% of the 741 patients in whom I performed coronary bypass surgery over this same period. All but 1 of these grafts were individual grafts (205 in situ grafts and 18 free grafts). One was a sequential graft. Anastomotic sites were comprised of 14 LADs (2 free grafts), 3 diagonal arteries (3 free grafts), 29 CX arteries (8 free grafts), and 178 RCAs (5 free grafts). The patients were 191 men and 32 women with an age range of 6 to 80 years (mean: 59 years). There were three cases (1%) of single-vessel disease, 24 cases (11%) of double-vessel disease, 165 cases (74%) of triple-vessel disease, and 31 cases (14%) of left main disease. There were 20 reoperations. As simultaneous operations, aortic valve replacement and mitral valve replacement were done for one case, left-ventricular aneurysmectomy and abdominal aorta replacement were conducted in two cases, lower-limb revascularization was done in five cases, cholecystectomy was simultaneously performed in ten cases, and splenectomy for associated idiopathic thrombocytopenic purpura was done in two cases. The mean number of distal anastomoses was 3.3, and the mean number for arterial grafts was 2.4. The ITA was combined with

Table 1
Gastroepiploic Artery Graft

Reported Results

Author	No. of Pts. (No. Redo.)	No. of RGEA in situ	No. of RGEA free	LAD	Diag.	Cx	RCA	Total	Patency	Early mortality
Carter[14]	30 (4)	30	0	0	0	35*		35†	7/9 (78%)	1 (3.3%)
Verkkala[16]	11 (?)	11	0	0	0	0	11	11	9/11 (82%)	0 (0%)
Mills[3]	39 (3)	26	15	0	5	4	34	43†	29/29 (100%)	3 (7.7%)
Lytle[17]	36 (22)	17	19	6*		8	22	36	9/9 (100%)	2 (5.6%)
Beretta[18]	20 (?)	0	20	4	1	13	9	27†	20/20 (100%)	0 (0%)
Pym[19]	57 (?)	56	1	0	0	5	52	57	25/26 (96%)	1 (1.8%)
Suma[23]	223 (20)	205	18	14	3	29	178	224†	161/170 (95%)	7 (3.1%)

Reported results of RGEA grafts. * Included bypass to circumflex (CX) artery and right coronary artery (RCA) in Carter's report and to left anterior descending (LAD) and diagonal artery in Lytle's report. † Included sequential RGEA grafts.

RGEA grafting in 215 cases (96%) (unilateral: 157 cases; bilateral: 58 cases). Recently, the IEA has been concomitantly used with increasing frequency.

The aortic crossclamp time, the cardiopulmonary bypass time, and the total surgical time have become shorter with the accumulation of experience as shown in Table 2.

Postoperative early deaths occurred in seven cases (3.1%). Four cases were due to cardiac failure, and one case each were due to renal failure, respiratory failure, and rupture of the abdominal aorta by an intra-aortic balloon catheter. Late deaths occurred in four cases: two cases were due to stroke, and one case each was due to renal failure and respiratory failure. A new Q wave was observed in four cases, and 98% of the cases were relieved from anginal symptoms. Postoperative early imaging was performed in 170 cases, and 161 RGEAs (95%) were found to be patent. Among those who underwent early postoperative angiography, the second angiography was performed in 43 cases at a mean of 2 years postoperatively (longest was 5 years), 41 RGEAs (95%) were patent and, thus, the midterm results of RGEAs were excellent (Fig. 16).[23]

Kusukawa et al.[24] have shown by stress myocardial scintigraphy that the in situ RGEA graft has sufficient flow capability under the maximal stress. The Thallium 201 washout rate significantly improved at the RGEA grafted area. Furthermore, in 11 patients who underwent sequential myocardial scintigraphy before and after surgery, the washout rate improved from $35 \pm 10\%$ preoperatively to $45 \pm 15\%$ early postsurgery and remained at $43 \pm 6\%$ and $48 \pm 15\%$ at 1 and 2 postoperative years, respectively.[23]

Table 2
**Gastroepiploic Artery Graft:
Duration of Surgery**

	1986–1989	1990	1991
Number of distal anastomoses	3.3	3.3	3.2
aortic crossclamp (min)	63.8	47.4	42.1
cardiopulmonary bypass (min)	112.9	92.7	72.5
total operation time (min)	343.2	291.9	254.6

Duration of surgery with RGEA grafts. Duration of aortic crossclamp, cardiopulmonary bypass, and total operation time has become shorter with experience. (from Suma H, et al.[23]).

GEA–RCA

A.K. 67F

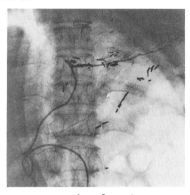 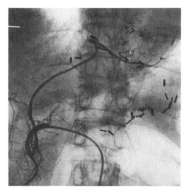

postop. 2 weeks   postop. 28 months

(A)

GEA–LAD

K.I. 54M

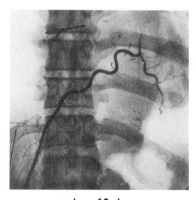 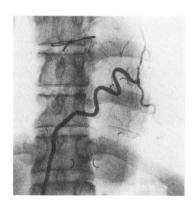

postop. 10 days   postop. 26 months

(B)

Fig. 16. Sequential postoperative angiograms of RGEA to the right coronary artery (RCA) (A) and to the left anterior descending artery (LAD) (B) during the early postoperative period and 2 years after surgery.

Basic Investigation

Histological study has shown less tendency of the RGEA to develop arteriosclerosis than do the coronary arteries, but it is not as resistant to arteriosclerosis as the ITA. Larsen et al.[25] demonstrated that significant arteriosclerosis was noted in only 7% of 102 gastroduodenal arteries, whereas it was found in 89% of 103 left coronary arteries in elderly people at autopsy. Suma and Takanashi[26] noted that the incidence of normal, mild, moderate, and severe pathological changes of RGEAs and ITAs taken from patients with severe coronary artery disease at the time of coronary bypass surgery were 46%, 43%, 9%, and 3% and 77%, 23%, 0%, and 0%, respectively.

The RGEA is a muscular artery that contains many smooth muscle cells in the media, whereas the ITA contains rich elastic fibers in the media. This difference in the medial component may play a role in which spasmogenecity between those two kinds of arteries is different and, thus, the tendency to develop foam cells from smooth muscle cells is higher in the RGEA.

Continuity of the internal elastic lamina is an important barrier in preventing the development of arteriosclerosis.[27] Although the ITA is known to have a strong continuity of the internal elastic lamina, the RGEA has a little more frequent fenestrations.[28]

Pharmacological response of the RGEA is different from the SV but similar to that of the ITA.[29] However, a recent study discovered a different response to histamine between the two arteries.[30,31] Histamine introduced contraction of the ITA but dilated the RGEA. The endothelium-derived relaxing factor (EDRF) may play an important role in this phenomenon.[31] We have demonstrated with a doppler flow study an increase of RGEA graft flow after a meal.[32] This reasonable organ-specific reaction of increased RGEA blood flow to the stomach during the digestive period seems to be a response to histamine released shortly after food ingestion. Thus, there is no concern that a meal-induced angina would produce a steal phenomenon.

The capability of prostacyclin production in the endothelium is another important point influencing graft patency. We have found that the RGEA produces more prostacyclin than the SV,[33] as was reported in the ITA.[34] To understand all the proper and important characteristics of the RGEA, further investigations are continuing at several institutes.

In summary, the RGEA in the past was an alternative conduit to be considered when other conduits were absent or could not be used.

With increasing usage and study, this conduit now is not only an alternative but also may be considered an important primary conduit for coronary revascularization. A big factor that could inhibit its usage, because of lack of experience in such situations at present, may be the question of how to handle this conduit (in situ) if it is patent in a patient who needs a redo coronary operation. If this becomes a problem in the future, perhaps the alternative method of free grafting will be needed with increasing frequency.

References

1. Bailey CP, Hirose T, Brancato R, Aventura A, et al. Revascularization of the posterior (diaphragmatic) portion of the heart. Ann Thorac Surg 1966; 791–805.
2. Vineberg A, Afridi S, Sahi S. Direct revascularization of acute myocardial infarction by implantation of left internal mammary artery into infarcted left ventricular myocardium. Surg Gyencol Obstet 1975; 140:44–52.
3. Mills NL, Everson CT. Right gastroepiploic artery: a third arterial conduit for coronary bypass. Ann Thorac Surg 1989; 47:706–711.
4. Hannoun L, Le Breton C, Bors V, Helenon C, et al. Radiological anatomy of the right gastroepiploic artery. Anat Clin 1984; 5:265–271.
5. Suma H, Fukumoto H, Takeuchi A. Coronary artery bypass grafting by utilizing in situ right gastroepiploic artery: basic study and clinical application. Ann Thorac Surg 1987; 44:394–397.
6. Saito T, Suma H, Terada Y, Wanibuchi Y, et al. Availability of the in situ right gastroepiploic artery for coronary artery bypass. Ann Thorac Surg 1992; 53:266–268.
7. Yamato T, Hamanaka Y, Hirata S, Sakai K. Esophagoplasty with an autogenous tubed gastric flap. Am J Surg 1979; 137:597– 602.
8. Van Son JAM, Smedts F, Vincent JG, Van Lier JH, et al. Comparative anatomic studies of various arterial conduits for myocardial revascularization. J Thorac Cardiovasc Surg 1990; 99:703–707.
9. Suma H, Wanibuchi Y, Furuta S, Isshiki T, et al. Comparative study between the gastroepiploic and the internal thoracic artery as a coronary bypass graft: size, flow, patency, histology. Eur J Cardio-thorac Surg 1991; 5:244–267.
10. Mills NL, Everson CT. Technical considerations for use of the gastroepiploic artery for coronary artery surgery. J Cardiac Surg 1989; 4:1–9.
11. Suma H. Coronary artery bypass grafting in patients with calcified ascending aorta: aortic no touch technique. Ann Thorac Surg 1989; 48:728–730.
12. Mills NL, Everson CT. Atherosclerosis of the ascending aorta and coronary artery bypass, pathology, clinical correlates, and operative management. J Thorac Cardiovasc Surg 1991; 102:546–553.
13. Pym J, Brown PM, Charrette EJP, Parker JO, et al. Gastroepiploic-coronary anastomosis: a viable alternative bypass graft. J Thorac Cardiovasc Surg 1987; 94:256–259.

14. Carter MJ. The use of the right gastroepiploic artery in coronary artery bypass grafting. Aust NZ J Surg 1987; 57:317– 321.
15. Attum AA. The use of the gastroepiploic artery for coronary artery bypass grafts: another alternative. Tex Heart Inst J 1987; 14:289–292.
16. Verkkala K, Jarvinen A, Keto P, Virtanen K, et al. Right gastroepiploic artery as a coronary bypass graft. Ann Thorac Surg 1989; 47:716–719.
17. Lytle BW, Cosgrove DM, Ratliff NB, Loop FD. Coronary artery bypass grafting with the right gastroepiploic artery. J Thorac Cardiovasc Surg 1989; 97:826–31.
18. Beretta L, Lemma M, Vanelli P, et al. Gastroepiploic artery free graft for coronary bypass. Eur J Cardio-thorac Surg 1990; 4:323–328.
19. Pym J, Parker JO, West RO. The right gastroepiploic artery as a coronary artery bypass graft. Abstract from 27th Annual Meeting of The Society of Thoracic Surgeons; 1990; San Francisco, Calif.:68.
20. Tanimoto Y, Matsuda Y, Masuda T, et al. Multiple free (aortocoronary) gastroepiploic artery grafting. Ann Thorac Surg 1990; 49:479–480.
21. Takeuchi Y, Gomi A, Okamura Y, Mori H, et al. Coronary revascularization in a child with Kawasaki disease: use of right gastroepiploic artery. Ann Thorac Surg 1990; 50:294–296.
22. Isomura T, Hisatomi K, Asoh S, et al. Revascularization with the right gastroepiploic artery in Kawasaki's disease. J Thorac Cardiovasc Surg 1990; 100:796–798.
23. Suma H, Wanibuchi Y, Terada Y, et al. The right gastroepiploic artery graft: clinical and angiographic midterm results in 200 patients. J Thorac Cardiovasc Surg 1993; 105:615–623.
24. Kusukawa J, Hirota Y, Kawamura K, et al. An assessment of the efficacy of aorta-coronary bypass surgery using gastroepiploic artery with thallium 201 myocardial scintigraphy. Circulation 1989; 80(suppl. I):135–140.
25. Larsen E, Johansen AA. Gastric arteriosclerosis in elderly people. Scand J Gastroenterol 1969; 4:387–389.
26. Suma H, Takanashi R. Arteriosclerosis of the gastroepiploic and internal thoracic arteries. Ann Thorac Surg 1990; 50:413–416.
27. Sims FH. A comparison of coronary and internal mammary arteries and implications of the results in the etiology of arteriosclerosis. Am Heart J 1990; 105:560–566.
28. Van Son JAM, Smedts F. Comparative study between the gastroepiploic and the internal thoracic artery as a coronary bypass graft. Eur J Cardiovasc Surg 1991; 5:505–507.
29. Koike R, Suma H, Kondo E, et al. Pharmacological response of internal mammary artery and gastroepiploic artery. Ann Thorac Surg 1990; 50:384–386.
30. O'Neil GS, Chest AH, Schyns CI, Tadjkarimi S, et al. Vascular reactivity of human internal mammary and gastroepiploic arteries. Ann Thorac Surg 1991; 52:1310–1314.
31. Ochiai M, Ohno M, Taguchi J, et al. Responses of human gastroepiploic arteries to vasoactive substances: differences to internal mammary arteries and saphenous veins. J Thorac Cardiovasc Surg 1992; 104:453–458.
32. Takayama T, Suma H, Wanibuchi Y. Physiological and pharmacological response of arterial graft flow after coronary artery bypass grafting mea-

sured with an implantable ultrasonic doppler miniprobe. Circulation 1992; 86(suppl. II):217–223.

33. Oku T, Yamane S, Suma H, et al. Comparison of prostacyclin production of human gastroepiploic artery and saphenous vein. Ann Thorac Surg 1990; 49:767–770.

34. Chaikhouni A, Crawford FA, Kochel PJ, Olanoff LS, et al. Human internal mammary artery produces more prostacyclin than saphenous vein. J Thorac Cardiovasc Surg 1986; 92:88–91.

Chapter 7

The Inferior Epigastric Artery

Charles Everson and Noel Mills

The internal mammary artery (IMA) terminates at approximately the seventh intercostal space, bifurcating into the musculophrenic artery and the superior epigastric artery, which courses down the abdominal wall, anastomosing with the inferior epigastric artery (IEA), a branch of the external iliac artery. The superiority of the IMA over the saphenous vein (SV) with respect to long-term patency when used for coronary artery grafting implies that vessels of similar character may also enjoy this superiority. Recently, there has developed an interest in and usage of the IEA in clinical applications based on this assumption. The first reported use of the IEA for coronary bypass was by Puig et al. in 1988,[1] with Vincent and associates[2] also reporting an early experience.

Anatomy

The IEA begins as a branch of the external iliac artery, arising from its medial side deep within the inguinal ligament. It then courses medially and superiorly between the transversalis fascia to become the largest artery on the abdominal wall. It travels on the deep surface of the rectus abdominous muscle, entering the rectus sheath anterior to the arcuate line to lie on the posterior rectus sheath for a variable distance. Along its course, the IEA supplies branches to

From Grooters RK and Nishida H: (editors): *Alternative Bypass Conduits and Methods for Surgical Coronary Revascularization.* © Futura Publishing Co., Inc., Armonk, NY, 1994.

the rectus muscle, gives rise to the external spermatic artery and a pubic branch, and terminally anastomoses with the superior epigastric artery. Two veins accompany the artery throughout its course, though they tend to have more numerous branches and form a single trunk prior to draining into the external iliac vein. The network created by the superior and inferior epigastric arteries supplies the anterior and medial aspect of the abdominal wall.

The position of the IEA within the rectus sheath is variable. It may remain on the posterior rectus sheath up to a level above the umbilicus prior to entering the muscle. It may enter the muscle below the umbilicus and travel in an intramuscular position until its anastomosis with the superior epigastric artery. Lastly, the IEA may be a bifurcated vessel with one limb remaining on the posterior sheath, the other entering the substance of the muscle. Each variation requires a different approach when the artery is harvested for surgical use. One limitation to the use of the IEA is its tendency to markedly decrease in internal diameter as it proceeds superiorly.

Histological studies reported by van Son et al.[3] reveal that the IEA is a muscular artery with only rare elastic lamella occurring in the media near its origin. This is in contrast to the IMA, which is classified as an elastic artery.

The absence of atherosclerotic disease in the IMA as compared to other arteries, most notably the coronary arteries, is presumed to some degree to be a result of the elastic content of the media of the IMA. The 4 to 15 elastic lamella in the media of the IMA have few discontinuities or fenestrations and may serve as a barrier to smooth-muscle migration into the media as an early event in atherosclerosis. This is opposed to the elastic membranes of the atherosclerotic-susceptible coronary arteries.

With respect to the degree of fenestration in the elastic tissue, the IEA is more similar to the IMA than it is to the coronary arteries when elastic tissue is present. Van Son et al.[4] found a gradual decrease in the elastic fibers in the IMA as it proceeded more distally. Therefore, although the IMA, the superior epigastric artery, and the IEA form an anatomical continuum, there is a marked histologic difference between that segment which is IMA and that which is the IEA—essentially the difference between an elastic versus a muscular artery. Whether this difference will confer different patency rates when the segments are used as coronary bypass grafts has, as yet, to be determined.

Surgical Technique

The left IEA, when harvested, is approached through a left-infraumbilical paramedian incision. The right IEA is approached in a mirror-image manner. The harvest of one IEA can be done simultaneously with the dissection of the IMA if a two-surgeon team is utilized. The anterior rectus sheath is opened longitudinally the length of the incision, and the underlying rectus muscle is dissected along its medial border and gently retracted laterally. Milgalter and Laks[5] alternatively describe the dissection of the lateral border of the rectus muscle from the sheath and medial retraction of the muscle for exposure of the vascular pedicle, though they postulate that the medial approach may better preserve the nerve supply to the muscle. The IEA is in an inferior position on the posterior rectus sheath with its two adjacent veins (Fig. 1). Individual branches are ligated with

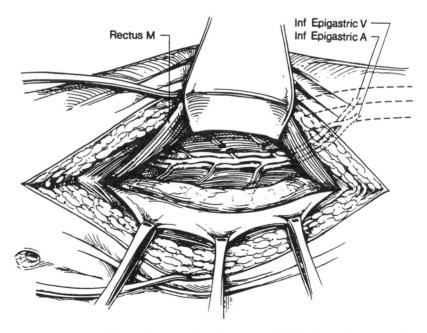

Rectus M

Inf Epigastric V
Inf Epigastric A

Fig. 1. Harvest of the inferior epigastric artery (IEA) is begun by retracting the rectus laterally after its fascia is opened directly anterior for the length of the incision. Undue traction on the rectus muscle (M) at this point can avulse penetrating branches (from Mills NL, et al.[6]).

4-0 silk and divided, with respect for the fragility of these small vessels, as the pedicle of the artery and surrounding veins is mobilized. Electrocautery is used to divide slips of the rectus muscle where necessary. The dissection proceeds inferiorly toward the origin of the IEA at the external iliac artery. The IEA will take a lateral and posterior course at this point, making exposure somewhat difficult. Vigorous retraction on the rectus muscle will be necessary, with care taken to avoid avulsion of side branches from the IEA as yet undivided. Pressing down on the peritoneum with a sponge stick aids in the exposure.

Early in our experience, a second incision in the groin was utilized to facilitate a division of the IEA at its origin, sometimes with a small divot of the parent vessel taken to facilitate the ultimate proximal anastomosis of the IEA to the aorta. Currently, neither is recommended.[6] The second incision has not proven necessary, and removing a piece of the wall of the external iliac artery is discouraged because of the liability of repairing a potentially atherosclerotic vessel at this point in the operation. Therefore, the IEA is suture-ligated near its origin with 2-0 silk, after individual ligation of its external spermatic and pubic branches. Barner at al.[7] note that the vas deferens passes adjacent and lateral to the IEA in this area. It potentially could be injured during this portion of the dissection, especially with division of the veins and artery near their origin. They advocate division of the vessels approximately 1 cm from the origin, with no diminution in the intraluminal size noted.

Once proximally divided, our technique is to cannulate the artery with a small olive-tipped needle and to infuse it with a heparinized PLASMALYTE solution (Baxter Healthcare Corp., Edwards Division, Irvine, Calif.). The dissection then continues superiorly or distally. At this point, variation may occur. If the vessels remain on the posterior rectus sheath, they may be easily mobilized with continued ligation of the side branches with 4-0 silk, producing a graft of very acceptable length. If, however, the vessel pierces and enters the rectus muscle, the dissection becomes more difficult. Careful tunneling and division of the muscle is necessary as the pedicle is pursued along its course. At some point, it may become more accessible to approach the vessels from the anterior surface of the muscle. As the dissection proceeds superiorly, it may be helpful to dissect the lateral border of the rectus muscle from the sheath and retract it medially. If the variant occurs where the IEA bifurcates below the level of the umbilicus, both limbs may be dissected if a Y-type graft can be utilized, though each limb will be small and the usable graft length shorter. The dissection is completed with suture ligation and transection of the pedicle.

Although the vessel produced is usually very acceptable for bypass grafting, Barner et al.[7] have reported 1 IEA in 37 patients that was pulseless and fibrotic. In the same report, 2 out of 14 IEAs revealed foci of calcification in the media on microscopic examination in a pattern suggestive of medial calcific sclerosis. This latter finding did not interfere with the luminal size or use of the vessel as a conduit. Milgalter and Laks[5] report that preoperative evaluation of the IEA is possible with the duplex scan (ultrasonic imaging and Doppler flow-signal analysis), tracing the IEA from the inguinal crease to the umbilicus along the lateral rectus border.

Once the vessel has been harvested, our practice has been to infuse it with a 1:40 dilution of body temperature papaverine-PLASMALYTE solution, to give mild dilation, and to check for hemostasis. A mark is placed along one border of the graft to aid in the avoidance of twists.

In 18 IEAs initially harvested by Mills et al.,[6] length ranged from 11.5 to 17 cm with proximal intraluminal diameters of 2.5 to 3.5 mm and distal internal diameters of 1.5 to 2.5 mm. Barner et al.,[7] with a total of 57 measured IEAs, found a mean length of 11.9 ± 2.6 cm and internal diameters of 2.0 ± 0.3 mm. Milgalter and Laks[5] report an average length of 11.4 ± 2.2 cm in 45 IEA grafts. Variants, in the IEA enters the rectus muscle or bifurcates within the sheath, produce grafts that are shorter with smaller distal diameters, which may place limits on the choice of vessels in the heart to which they can be grafted.

Some care must be given to the closure of the abdominal wound. Although rectus muscle or abdominal wall necrosis remains a concern, especially with the bilateral IEA harvest,[8] this has not occurred in our experience. The use of a Jackson-Pratt type drain is encouraged. Complications limited to abdominal wound drainage, superficial wound infection, and fat necrosis requiring wound healing by secondary intention have been reported.[5–7] All reported problems to date have been in obese, often diabetic, patients. Hernias and dysfunction of the rectus muscle have not been reported.

Anastomoses

The handling characteristics of the IEA in construction of the distal, coronary anastomosis are similar to those of the IMA, though

Barner[7] has noted that there is a lesser tendency for the IEA to split into two layers as can occur with the IMA. The anastomotic techniques are similar. Our practice involves a 5–6 mm coronary arteriotomy and construction of a running 8-0 prolene suture line, proceeding from heel to toe and back halfway. Three-way patency is demonstrated, and the graft is de-aired prior to securing the anastomosis. The graft is then tacked to the epicardium in several sites with 5-0 prolene to prevent tension on the suture line and to prevent the formation of twists.

A somewhat controversial aspect of the use of the IEA is the coronary artery to which the graft is placed. The short graft length limits the reach of the IEA if an aortic proximal anastomosis is planned. Although some groups have been reluctant to use the IEA for the left anterior descending (LAD) or right coronary artery (RCA) systems, employing it instead for more minor branches such as the diagonal, others have used the IEA for the more primary vessels.[6,7] Combined data from 3 reported series reveal the following vessels, or arteries, grafted (total: 112, including sequential and Y grafts): obtuse marginal—33, diagonal—29, ramus intermedius—13, RCA—7, posterior descending artery—1, posterior lateral artery—6, and LAD—22.[5–7] As noted by van Son,[3] the as yet established long-term patency of the IEA may encourage a more limited use to smaller, secondary target vessels until data have defined these characteristics.

The proximal anastomosis of the IEA may be approached in a variety of ways. If it is of sufficient length, the proximal IEA may be anastomosed directly to a nonpathological ascending aorta via a 4 mm punch site, using a 6-0 Prolene (Ethicon Endo-Surgery, Cincinnati, Ohio) on a BV-1 needle in a manner similar to a free IMA graft (Fig. 2). If possible, it is helpful to spatulate the IEA by opening it through one of its larger branches, either the external spermatic or pubic artery. It is always desirable to demonstrate the patency of the proximal anastomosis by passing on an appropriately sized probe via another aortotomy site, if one is present. Alternatives that are useful in a diseased aorta include anastomosis of the IEA to a SV graft end-to-side or placement of a pericardial or vein patch to the aortotomy site, with subsequent anastomosis of the IEA to the patch. On early postoperative angiography, Puig et al.[9] noted 100% patency of IEAs anastomosed to either SV or bovine pericardial patches, versus 2 out of 8 grafts that were directly anastomosed to the aorta and were obstructed.

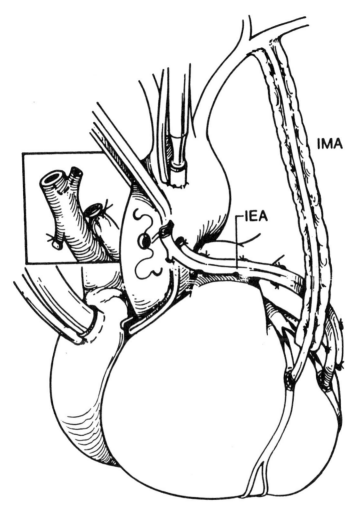

Fig. 2. The inferior epigastric artery (IEA) has been opened across a side branch to make the "mouth" larger for the proximal anastomosis. That anastomosis is performed using a 6-0 polypropylene suture on a BV-1 needle (from Mills NL, et al.[6]).

The alternative for an IEA that is too short for an aortic anastomosis is to place it end-to-side to another conduit, either a SV or an IMA. With careful planning and measurement, the IEA can be anastomosed to the IMA prior to initiation of extracorporeal circulation to create an artificial arterial Y graft. Such an anastomosis is performed after demonstration of the adequacy of flow in the IMA (150 cc/min minimal) and is constructed of either 7-0 or 8-0 Prolene, with care taken to demonstrate three-way patency prior to securing the anastomosis.

An interesting concept presented by Mills et al.[8] is the recommendation that the vein accompanying the IEA also be anastomosed to the mammary vein to create a true pedicle graft. The attempt here is to relieve the venous engorgement in the IEA pedicle, which may have consequences on postoperative patency.

Comment

The great hindrance in evaluating the IEA is the lack of both a substantial number of early angiographic results and any long-term studies. Clinical results, based on patient outcome, are of little benefit because, at best, the IEA is contributing only two and, more frequently, one graft in a multiple-graft revascularization. Puig and associates[9] report an 85% (151.7) patency rate at early angiography (8–10 days postoperatively). Our experience with 8 patients studied up to 10 months postoperatively was less favorable, with 3 widely patent grafts, 2 closed grafts, and the remaining 3 grafts patent, with diffuse narrowing compatible with arterial spasm. Barner et al.[7] wisely question the appropriateness of the IEA graft in patients in whom good SV is available. There are no angiographic studies as yet that demonstrate a comparable, much less superior, patency for the IEA graft over the SV.

Very recent studies reported by Massa et al.[10] have questioned whether all free arterial grafts are susceptible to failure because of spasm. Their experimental findings indicate a hypercontractility (spasm), with an increased sensitivity to catecholamines in free arterial grafts. Additional reports of favorable control of arterial spasm with calcium channel blockers, such as diltiazem, offer hope that this problem may be correctable. Renewed interest in the radial artery (RA) free graft (Chapter 8) is based on this possibility; perhaps a reassessment of the IEA in a similar manner is warranted. At the present time, the IEA remains an alternative graft to be considered in patients in whom adequate SV is not available, after better-studied and proven IMAs and right gastroepiploic arteries (RGEAs) have been utilized. Although the IEA can be harvested without significant increased morbidity or mortality, its efficacy in coronary revascular-ization remains unproven.

References

1. Puig LB, Ciongoli W, Cividanes GVD, et al. Ateria epigastrica inferior como enxerto livre. Uma nova alternativa na revascularizaco do miocar-dio. Arz Bras Cardiol 1988; 50:259.
2. Vincent JG, van Son JAM, Skotnicki SH. Inferior epigastric artery as a conduit in myocardial revascularization: the alternative free arterial graft. Ann Thorac Surg 1990; 49:323–325.
3. van Son JAM. Histology of the internal mammary artery versus the in-ferior epigastric artery. Letter to Ann Thorac Surg 1992; 53:1147–1149.
4. van Son JAM, Smedts F, Vincent JG, et al. Comparative anatomic studies of various arterial conduits for myocardial revascularization. J Thorac Surg 1990; 99:703–707.
5. Milgalter E, Laks H. A technique to harvest the inferior epigastric arter-ies for coronary bypass procedures. J Cardiovasc Surg 1991; 6:306–310.
6. Mills NL, Everson CT. Technique for use of the inferior epigastric artery as a coronary bypass graft. Ann Thorac Surg 1991; 51:208–214.
7. Barner HB, Naunheim KS, Fiore AC, et al. Use of the inferior epigastric artery as a free graft for myocardial revascularization. Presented at the Society of Thoracic Surgeons, 1991.
8. Mills NL, Everson CT, Hockmuth DR. Free arterial grafts. Curr Opinion Cardiol 1991; 6:898–903.
9. Puig LB, Ciongolli W, Cividanes GVL, et al. Inferior epigastric artery as a free graft for myocardial revascularization. J Thorac Surg 1990; 99:251–255.
10. Massa G, Johansson S, Kimblad PO, et al. Might free arterial grafts fail due to spasm? Ann Thorac Surg 1991; 51:94–101.

8

The Radial Artery

Ronald K. Grooters and Hiroshi Nishida

The radial artery (RA) initially appeared to be one of the ideal conduits for coronary artery bypass grafting (CABG). The size of the RA is nearly the same as the coronary artery, whereas the saphenous vein (SV) is disproportionately large. In theory, the RA should have been superior because it offers a graft with elasticity and a regular lumen that provides physiological flow when compared to the SV, a conduit fixed in diameter with valves present. Additionally, the RA is long, has an ideal diameter, is tougher when compared to the internal mammary artery (IMA), and it is generally easier to harvest and suture. Although the early investigators, Carpentier et al.,[1] Curtis et al.,[2] Fisk et al.,[3] Grondin,[4] and others (Table 1) observed spasticity of the RA graft, they noted excellent immediate patency rates. It was the intermediate patency rates (1 month to 1 year) that were unacceptable. Until recently,[5,6] the RA had been completely avoided as a conduit for myocardial revascularization.

Comparative Anatomical and Histologic Characteristics

Acar and colleagues[5] recently compared the microscopic and anatomical features of the RA to the IMA in 30 patients undergoing CABG and in ten fresh cadavers. Both arteries were dilated using a papaverine solution and measured. Segments of these arteries were also fixed in 3% formaldehyde solution for histologic and morphometric study. The 30 surgical patients were angiographically studied at 2 weeks postoperatively.

From Grooters RK and Nishida H: (editors): *Alternative Bypass Conduits and Methods for Surgical Coronary Revascularization.* © Futura Publishing Co., Inc., Armonk, NY, 1994.

Table 1
Radial Artery in Aortocoronary Grafting

Center	Patients	Grafts	Early Patency	Late Patency (M)
Montreal Heart Institute (Montreal)	12	17	85.0%	25.0% (14)
Callaghan (Edmonton)	37	48	71.5%	50.0% (4)
Curtis (Nashville)	79	92	100.0%	45.3% (4)
Carpentier (Paris)	30	40	100.0% (0–10 m)	<33.0% (12–15)
Edwards (Albuquerque)	—	30	—	<50.0% (9)
Loop (Cleveland)	14	16	—	42.0% (6)

From Grondin P.[4]
M: months postoperatively

Results

In the RA, the length and diameter were greater, and the richness of planimetry collateral branches was more abundant (Table 2). Morphometric measurements for the thickness of the intima and media were significantly higher in the RA when compared to the IMA. Microscopic analysis also revealed that this increased wall thickness was derived from all three layers (intima, media, and adventitia). The intima of the RA contained multiple layers of subendothelial cells beneath a single endothelial layer. The internal elastic lamina was the same for both vessels. Major differences in the media existed. The RA media contained myocytes organized in multiple tight layers with scant amounts of connective tissue. The IMA myocytes were larger and irregular with a loose structure of elastic fibers and ground substance. The external elastic lamina was identical in both arteries. The adventitia layer, containing the vasa vasorum, nerves, and lymphatic vessels, was thicker in the RA. Angiograms 2 weeks postoperatively revealed all grafts to be patent, but in four RA grafts narrowing was present. Narrowing disappeared in one patient following in situ injection with nitroglycerin. Late angiograms (12

Table 2
**Anatomical Characteristics of the Radial Artery
and the Internal Mammary Artery**

	Radial Artery	Internal Mammary Artery
Length (cm)	22.5 + 1.2	19.2 + 0.8
Diameter (mm)	2.7 + 0.06	1.9 + 0.07
Richness in collateral branches	+ + +	+
Parietal thickness		
(intima + media) mm²	3.30 + 0.04	2.39 + 0.21

Adapted from Acer C, et al.[5]

months after surgery) in two patients with previous abnormalities were normal. The other RA grafts that were normal on the first angiogram remained normal, as did all the compared IMA grafts.

Expanded Clinical Study

This clinical study was expanded to include 104 patients using 122 RA grafts and was reported by Acar and associates.[6] Left IMA grafts were concomitantly used as in situ grafts in 100 patients, and right IMA grafts were used as in situ grafts in 19 patients; either IMA was used as a free graft in 29 patients. The SV was also used in 24 of the patients. A mean of 2.8 grafts per patient was performed. One patient died, and two patients sustained perioperative myocardial infarctions. No ischemia of the hand developed. The techniques of harvesting and handling the RA were postulated to be very important changes from 20 years ago.

Technique of Harvest

Prior to the harvest of the RA, an Allen's test and Doppler studies of the forearm were done. The incision was made directly over the RA from the wrist to the elbow. The antebrachial fascia was divided, and the RA was removed as a pedicle including the satellite veins and surrounding tissue. Collateral branches were ligated with clips. The RA was dissected from the pulse groove to the proximal segment lying beneath the brachio radialis up to the humeral bifurcation. These muscles were retracted, not divided. Once mobilized, the pedicle was wrapped in a papaverine-soaked sponge and not removed until cardiopulmonary bypass was started.

Before its use, the RA was hydrostatically dilated by using a blood and papaverine (40 mg/L) solution until the spasm was totally relieved. No intraluminal instrumentation, such as probe dilatation, was used. The arteries were sutured with 7-0 or 8-0 polypropylene.

Angiographic Results

The patency rate for the first 56 RA grafts studied 3 weeks after operation was 100%. Segmental narrowing was noted in six patients, moderate narrowing in four, and severe narrowing in two. Three of these lesions regressed with intragraft vasodilation and Ca^{++} blocking agents, but in three RA grafts the lesions remained.

The in situ IMA grafts were all patent at 3 weeks, but 2 of the 18 free IMA grafts were occluded, and 2 other grafts had a "string sign" for an early patency rate of 77.8%. Eight of nine vein grafts were patent (88.9%).

Repeat angiograms 6–13 months postoperatively (9.2 months average) demonstrated 29 of 31 RA grafts (93.5%) to be patent. Only one graft had a moderate stenosis, which was at the distal anastomosis. Two other grafts with previous stenoses were normal at 12 months. The late patency rate for the in situ IMA grafts was 100% and 69.3% for the free IMA grafts.

Discussion

The graft failure of the RA experienced 20 years ago was thought to be due first to fibrointimal hyperplasia and second to the intense spasticity of this "muscular artery." This spasm may have been easily induced by mechanical dilatation from the use of intraluminal probes and direct instrumentation during harvest that resulted in a skeletonized RA, leaving it without its satellite veins and vasa vasorum.

To demonstrate this effect, Chiu[7] demonstrated in a canine experiment that disrupting the vasa vasorum in "muscular" arteries such as the RA and then preventing vasa vasorum regeneration by wrapping the grafts in a plastic sheet enhanced the severity of subintimal hyperplasia. In the two dogs killed early after operation, the wrapped arterial grafts showed subintimal and medial necrosis with leukocyte infiltration.

This ischemia or necrosis associated with an absence of blood supply from important surrounding nutrient vessels used as grafts is likely to contribute to the etiology of graft failure. This may be prevented by using a harvest technique that preserves this perivascular tissue. In rethinking the cause of RA graft failure,[6] it can now be postulated that the RA must be dissected as a pedicle with surrounding tissue to include its accompanying veins; then with a solution of blood and papaverine the RA graft must be gently dilated with hydrostatic pressure. This will hopefully prevent the ischemia and mechanical damage that induce the causative factors (persistent spasm and intense intimal hyperplasia) of early graft failure. The use of Ca^{++} blocking agents intraoperatively and long-term postoperatively is also thought to be important in preventing spasm.

Carpentier et al.[1] concluded years ago that unless the spasticity of the RA was controlled, the conduit should not be used for coronary artery grafting. If this limiting factor is prevented, this conduit may be an ideal graft if we consider that (1) the RA, like most upper-extremity arteries, may rarely be affected by atherosclerosis; (2) this graft is from a systemic pressure environment; (3) the diameter of the RA approximates that of the most important coronary arteries; (4) the length (20 cm or more) will reach most distal coronary vessels; and (5) the wall of the RA is durable and tough, an ideal technical consideration for the construction of both the proximal and distal anastomosis. Since this better understanding of the pathogenesis and treatment of RA graft spasm improves the short-term patency rate (1 year or less), long-term studies are now needed to determine this conduit's place in the spectrum of conduits available for myocardial revascularization. The RA may finally end up as a very satisfactory alternative to the venous conduits and perhaps some arterial conduits.

References

1. Carpentier A, Guermonprez JL, Deloche A, Frechette C, et al. The aorto-to-coronary radial artery bypass graft. Ann Thorac Surg 1973; 16:111–121.
2. Curtis JJ, Stoney WS, Alford Jr WB, Burrus GR, et al. Intimal hyperplasia: a cause of radial artery aortocoronary bypass graft failure. Ann Thorac Surg 1975; 20:628–635.
3. Fisk RL, Brooks CH, Callaghan JC, Cvorkin J. Experience with the radial artery graft for coronary artery bypass. Ann Thorac Surg 1976; 21:513–518.

4. Grondin P. Small diameter arteries in the aortocoronary position. In: Sawyer P and Kaplitt MJ, eds. Vascular Grafts. New York: Appleton-Century-Crofts, 1978.
5. Acar C, Jebara VA, Portoghese M, Fontaliran F, et al. Comparative anatomy and histology of the radial artery and the internal thoracic artery: implication for coronary artery bypass. Surg Radiol Anat 1991; 13:283–288.
6. Acar C, Jebara VA, Portoghese M, Beyssen B, et al. Revival of the radial artery for coronary artery bypass grafting. Ann Thorac Surg 1992; 54:652–660.
7. Chiu CJ. Why do radial artery grafts for aortocoronary bypass fail? A reappraisal. Ann Thorac Surg 1976; 22:520–523.

9

The Splenic Artery

Ronald K. Grooters and Hiroshi Nishida

This chapter is mainly a history of the splenic artery used as a bypass conduit to the coronary arteries, primarily the right coronary artery (RCA). The splenic artery was considered to be an alternative conduit, but no recent studies of its usage to revascularize the heart have been reported or repeated. Long-term follow-up angiographic studies (greater than 2 years) cannot be found in the literature. Yet, it appears that intermediate patency rates of this conduit are just as good as and may be better than those for the saphenous vein (SV). Maybe we should not totally discard consideration of this conduit.

History

In 1973, Edwards and his colleagues[1] reported on their efforts to use the splenic artery for coronary revascularization. It was speculated that arterial in situ grafts, including splenic artery grafts, would be better than SVs and, additionally, that the splenic artery could easily reach a coronary artery on the back of the heart. Mueller et al.[2] angiographically studied six splenic artery grafts 2 weeks after coronary bypass and found five to be patent. Grondin[3] reported that a later study by Edwards showed that 90% of the splenic grafts were angiographically patent 1 to 2 years later, which was comparable to if not better than the patency rate for SV grafts for that time period. Difficulties in harvesting and handling the splenic artery, its tortuosity, the increased frequency of atherosclerosis, and the frequent need for

From Grooters RK and Nishida H: (editors): *Alternative Bypass Conduits and Methods for Surgical Coronary Revascularization.* © Futura Publishing Co., Inc., Armonk, NY, 1994.

splenectomy, in spite of very good intermediate patency rates, caused surgeons to lose their enthusiasm for this artery as a coronary artery graft.

Technique

As Edwards et al.[1] reported, all operations were performed through a sternal-splitting incision, which was then extended 4–5 cm toward the umbilicus for easy entry into the peritoneal cavity. The lesser omental sac between the stomach and the colon was entered by dividing the gastric colic ligament to the splenic flexure of the colon. The splenic artery was usually visible, emerging from behind the pancreas at the junction of the body and tail. Dissection was begun at that point and extended proximally to the celiac axis, as well as distally to the hilum of the spleen. Many small branches to the body of the pancreas had to be ligated. Approximately 15 cm of the splenic artery was exposed and then was ligated distally and divided. The spleen was not removed at first but, because splenic infarcts developed, removal of the spleen was later necessary. Some splenic arteries were quite tortuous and redundant, requiring that fibrous bands between loops in the artery be carefully divided. This straightened the artery and prevented obstructive kinks, and at the same time it helped lengthen the artery.

The divided artery was then passed behind the stomach through a 2 cm incision in the membranous portion of the diaphragm into the pericardial cavity (Fig. 1). Occasionally, to facilitate passing the graft through the diaphragm, the triangular ligament of the liver was divided, and the 2 cm hole in the diaphragm was stretched with the index finger to prevent compression of the splenic artery as it passed through. The opening in the diaphragm was located directly opposite the RCA, usually just proximal to the posterior descending branch.

After cardiopulmonary bypass was established and the patient was cooled to 28°C, the aorta was crossclamped for periods up to 20 minutes. A longitudinal incision was made in the distal RCA or in the posterior descending branch. The beveled end of the splenic artery was then sutured to the coronary artery using a 6-0 continuous synthetic suture. The splenic artery graft was attached to the coronary artery in either a retrograde or an antegrade fashion, what-

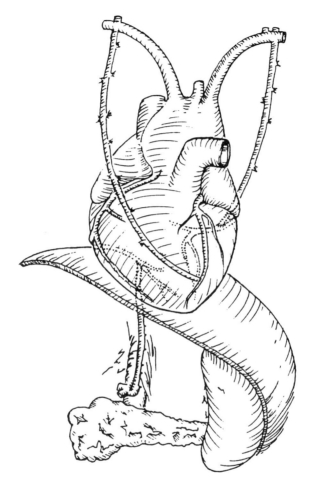

Fig. 1. Triple coronary bypass is performed with the splenic artery for the right artery, the left mammary artery for the circumflex artery, and the right mammary artery for obstruction of the LAD (from Edwards WS, et al.[1]).

ever way allowed the graft to lie most naturally to prevent kinking. The internal mammary arteries (IMAs) were used (Fig. 1) at the same time to revascularize the left anterior descending (LAD) and/or the circumflex (CX) arteries. All the arterial grafts were used as in situ grafts.

Pathology

The splenic artery is a very "serpentine" artery with fibrous bands between loops. It has also been found to be a friable artery, with its layers easily separated by surgical manipulation. Both of these tendencies require a very meticulous touch during its use as a conduit, more so than the IMA. The most discouraging feature was the frequency of atherosclerosis as determined by Larsen[4] in a study of 103 autopsied patients 60 years of age or older. He found that 96.4% (89 out of 103 patients) had significant coronary atherosclerosis, but 42.7% (44 of the 103) of these patients also had advanced atherosclerotic lesions in their splenic arteries. Although the splenic artery seems to have atherosclerotic lesions 50% less often than the coronary arteries, this tendency is significantly worse than that of the IMA in which atherosclerosis is rarely found (Chapter 1) and also the right gastroepiploic artery (RGEA) (Chapter 6).

Conclusion

Although the use of the splenic artery is mostly historical, we still have to keep in mind that this graft is as good as, if not better than, the SV when comparing both immediate and intermediate patency rates. As an alternative conduit, if other choices are not available and a surgeon wants to overcome the technical difficulties of harvesting and preparing the graft, this artery could conceivably be an option for coronary revascularization. We know that this may still be controversial.

References

1. Edwards WS, Blakely WR, Lewis CE. Technique of coronary bypass with autogenous arteries. J Thorac Cardiovasc Surg 1973; 65(2):272–275.
2. Mueller CF, Lewis CE, Edwards WS. The angiographic appearance of splenic-to-coronary artery anastomosis. Radiology 1973; 106:513–516.
3. Grondin P. Small diameter arteries in the aortocoronary position. In: Sawyer P and Kaplitt MJ, eds. Vascular Grafts. New York, NY: Appleton-Century-Crofts, 1978: 375–377.
4. Larsen E, Johansen A, Andersen D. Gastric arteriosclerosis in elderly people. Scand J Gastroenterol 1969; 4:387–389.

10

The Subclavian Artery

Ronald K. Grooters and Hiroshi Nishida

A left subclavian-coronary artery (LSCA) grafting for an anomalous origin of the left coronary artery from the pulmonary artery (ALCAPA) was first attempted by Apley et al.[1] in 1957. The procedure was unsuccessful. Myer et al.,[2] in 1968, were the first to report a successful in situ subclavian-coronary artery bypass in a four-month-old patient without the use of cardiopulmonary bypass (CPB). Pinsky et al.[3] successfully used CPB with hypothermia for a subclavian-coronary artery bypass, but other case reports have shown that CPB is not always necessary.[4-9] The LSCA can also be used as a free graft from the posterior aspect of the ascending aorta via the transverse sinus to the left main coronary[10-13] with excellent long-term results. Arciniegas et al.,[11] in two patients, and Backer et al.,[14] in one patient, successfully brought the free graft through the pulmonary artery in a procedure similar to that of Takeuchi et al.[15] Doty et al.[16] have even used the right subclavian artery to construct an anastomosis to the left coronary artery originating from the right pulmonary artery (Fig. 1). The left subclavian has also been used by Suzuki et al.[17] as a graft to the left anterior descending (LAD) for a patient with Bland-White-Garland syndrome. CPB was needed, and a patent ductus ligation was also required.

Initially, ligation of the left coronary artery at its pulmonary artery origin was the most widely used technique,[18] but the review by Likar et al.[19] showed that mortality was high (11 out of 27 patients) with ligation. The 11 deaths were in patients under the age of 18 months. Satisfactory results have also been reported[20-22] when a saphenous vein (SV) aortocoronary bypass was used for

From Grooters RK and Nishida H: (editors): *Alternative Bypass Conduits and Methods for Surgical Coronary Revascularization.* © Futura Publishing Co., Inc., Armonk, NY, 1994.

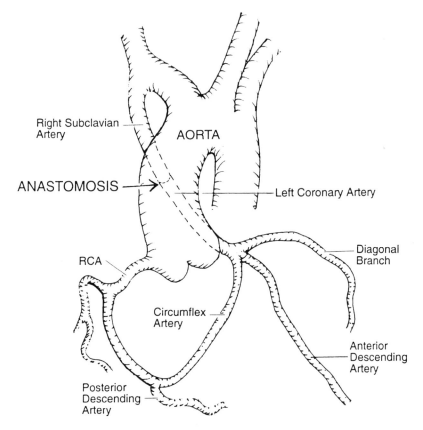

Fig. 1. Postoperative coronary angiogram (composite tracing). Two-coronary artery sytem with left coronary artery filled via right subclavian artery (from Doty DB, et al.[16]).

ALCAPA, but this alternative may not produce the same short- and long-term results because of the occlusive problems noted for venous conduits.

Kitamura and colleagues[23] have also demonstrated angiographically that the vein graft does not grow with the pediatric patient. Direct anastomosis of the left main coronary artery to the ascending aorta is also possible in some patients,[10,12] but only if the anomalous coronary artery originates from the posterior aspect of the pulmonary artery. A graft is needed in most patients to correct on

ALCAPA, and the subclavian artery-coronary artery grafting is most often the alternative operation of choice.

Technique

The left subclavian-left coronary artery graft is easily accomplished via a left posterolateral thoracotomy without CPB. It is a good idea to harvest or at least expose a segment of the SV prior to the thoracotomy in case the subclavian artery cannot be used as a conduit or is too short. The chest is entered through the fourth intercostal space. The subclavian artery is dissected from its origin to the thoracic outlet. Vertebral arteries and internal mammary arteries (IMAs) are individually ligated. Once mobilized and transected, the distal end is brought to the position of the left coronary origin to see if the grafting can be done without tension and kinking. The trunk of the left main coronary artery, usually arising from the posterolateral surface of the pulmonary artery, is exposed. This initially may require some careful dissection of the pulmonary artery proximally and the left main coronary artery distally. Other collateral vessels frequently need ligating to facilitate exposure and mobilization of the left main trunk.

Before transection of the left main coronary artery, it is occluded to determine if perfusion of the myocardium is adequate as reflected by electrocardiographic changes or hemodynamic decompensation. If the patient remains stable, the operation can proceed without CPB. The end-to-end (distal end of the subclavian artery to the orifice of the left main coronary artery) is the preferred technique (Fig. 2). This can only be done if the pulmonary artery can be side clamped so that a button of the pulmonary artery can be included with the origin of the left main coronary artery.

The pulmonary artery is oversewn with 4-0 or 5-0 polypropylene suture, and the graft anastomosis is sutured with a continuous 6-0 or 7-0 polypropylene suture. The end-to-side (left subclavian to left main coronary artery) technique with ligation of the left main trunk is also satisfactory, and the left subclavian to the anterior descending coronary artery technique is possible[7] but may require CPB. The subclavian and coronary artery clamps are removed, and hemostasis is established. CPB should be available and could be used either as a femoral-femoral bypass or a left pulmonary artery-descending aorta bypass circuit.

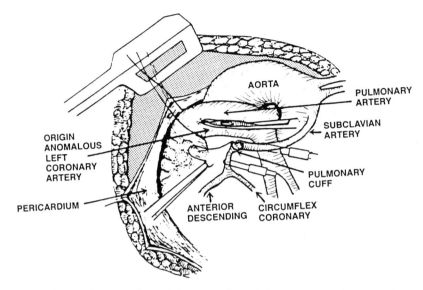

Fig. 2. Surgical approach via left posterolateral thoracotomy. The anomalous coronary artery is detached from the pulmonary artery with a cuff of vessel wall and anastomosed end-to-end to the left subclavian artery through a left thoracotomy (from Senderoff E, at al.[5]).

Free Graft Techniques

Retroaortic Aortocoronary Bypass Grafting

Arciniegas et al.[11] and Neches et al.[10] described the use of a free segment of the left subclavian artery exposed through a midsternotomy and dissected extrapleurally. It was then transected at both the apex of the chest and at its aortic origin. This graft was anastomosed to the posterior wall of the ascending aorta and then passed through the transverse sinus of the pericardium to be sutured to the left main coronary artery, end-to-side (Fig. 3). The ostium of the ALCAPA was closed by directed suture through a pulmonary arteriotomy.

Transpulmonary Aortocoronary Bypass Grafting

If the length of the free subclavian artery segment appears too short or the left main coronary artery is very small, the transpulmonary arterial adaptation described by Arciniegas et al.[11] may be very

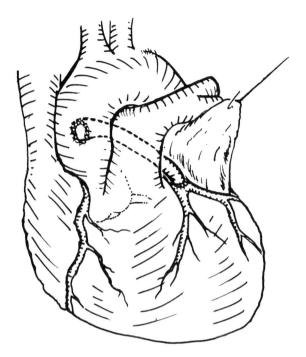

Fig. 3. Illustration of retroaortic aortocoronary bypass grafting with a free segment of the left subclavian coronary artery. The graft passes through the transverse sinus of the pericardium and is anastomosed to the left main coronary artery (from Arciniegas E, et al.[11]).

useful (Fig. 4). This allows for better exposure and easier construction of all vascular anastomoses. First, a 4 mm circular aortopulmonary "window" is constructed, and then with the main pulmonary artery open, one end of the subclavian artery graft is sutured around the aortopulmonary anastomosis, and the other end is sutured about the ostium of the anomalous left coronary artery (Fig. 4a). The pulmonary artery is widened with a small pericardial patch to avoid any potential narrowing of its lumen by the intrapulmonary artery free subclavian graft (Fig. 4b). Interrupted 7-0 polypropylene sutures are used to construct all the anastomoses during periods of hypothermic circulatory arrest. This is a modification of the Takeuchi procedure, which reconstituted a flap of the anterior pulmonary artery wall as the intrapulmonary conduit from the ascending aorta to the left main coronary artery.[15]

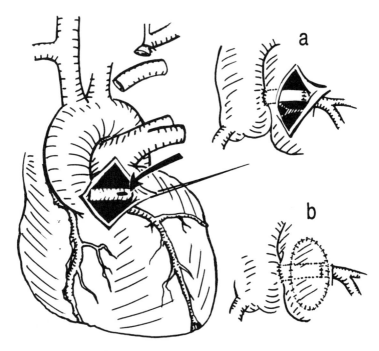

Fig. 4. Illustration of transpulmonary arterial aortocoronary bypass grafting with a free segment of the left subclavian-coronary artery (LSCA). Left: a 4 mm aortopulmonary "window" is constructed; (top right: a) the LSCA segment is sutured, within the pulmonary artery, to the aortopulmonary anastomosis and around the ostium of the anomalous left coronary artery; (bottom right: b) pericardial patch angioplasty prevents luminal compromise of the pulmonary artery (from Arciniegas E, et al.[11]).

Results

Within the first 3 months of surgery, clinical improvement has been observed by most authors. The cardiac silhouette on chest X rays has decreased in size. The median sternotomy approach using CPB and hypothermia has been equally as successful as the posterolateral approach without CPB. The two most-frequent factors responsible for operative deaths are preoperative severe ventricular dysfunction with congestive heart failure and mitral insufficiency.[13] Long-term follow-up (4–10 years) of the survivors using stress testing demonstrates improvement in exercise tolerance in most patients. Of the angiographic studies done on surviving patients (Table 1),

Table 1

Reports of the Subclavian Artery Used as a Coronary Artery Bypass

Author/ Year Reported	No. Patients/ Patient Age	Condition	Operative Technique	Outcome
Apley[1] 1957	1 patient/ 11 mos	ALCAPA*	LS to LCA**; no pump	unsuccessful
Myer[2] 1968	1 patient/ 4 mos	ALCAPA	LS to LCA; no pump	alive & well at 10 mos
Pinsky[3] 1973	2 patients/ 4 mos & 8 ½ mos.	ALCAPA	LS to LCA; CPB[x] with hypothermia	alive & well
Neches[10] 1974	2 patients/ 7 mos & 5 yrs	ALCAPA	1–LS to LCA; no pump 1–free graft; CPB with deep hypothermia	alive & well; both patent
Horiuchi[4] 1975	1 patient/ 5 mos	ALCAPA	LS to LCA; CPB used	alive & well 8 mos postop
Doty[16] 1976	1 patient/ 10 mos	ALCARPA°	RS to LCA°°; no pump	graft patent 4 mos postop
Senderoff[5] 1976	1 patient/ 5 ys	ALCAPA	LS to LCA; no pump	graft patent 3 mos postop
Suzuki[17] 1978	1 patient/ 6 mos	B-W-G[+]	LS to LCA; PDA[xx] ligated; CPB used	alive with mitral insufficiency 26 mos postop
Monro[6] 1978	1 patient/ 6 mos	ALCAPA	LS to LCA; no pump	graft patent 22 mos postop
Yoshida[7] 1980	1 patient 3 ½ yrs	ALCAPA	LS to LAD; CPB used	alive & well 5 yrs postop
Champsaur[8] 1980	3 patients/ 3–30 mos	ALCAPA	LS to LCA; no pump	alive & well
Arciniegas[11] 1980	7 patients/ 5 pts: 5–11 mos/ 2 pts: 3 & 4 mos	ALCAPA	5–retro-aortic ACBG[a] (CPB) free graft/ 2–TPLSCA[aa] graft (CPB) free graft	alive & well; one graft occlusion alive & well 3.5–7.5 ys

Table 1
(continued)

Author/ Year Reported	No. Patients/ Patient Age	Condition	Operative Technique	Outcome
Sanderson[12] 1981	3 patients/ 7 & 9 yrs	ALCAPA	2–in situ LS to LCA; 1–free graft ACBG*	alive & well 4 & 7 yrs; alive & well 7 yrs
Laborde[13] 1981	9 patients/ 4 mos to 9 yrs	ALCAPA	9 free graft ACBG*	4 operative deaths; 5 alive & well
Montigny[9] 1990	4 patients/ 27–44 mos	ALCAPA	4–in situ LS to LCA; no pump	all grafts patent 6–46 mos
Backer[14] 1992	5 patients/ 2–19 mos	ALCAPA	5–in situ LS to LCA; no pump	alive & well at 4–10 yrs with 1 anastomosis stenotic

ALCAPA* anomalous origin of the left coronary artery from the pulmonary artery; LS to LCA** left subclavian artery graft to left coronary artery; B-W-G + Bland-White-Garland syndrome; CPB^x cardiopulmonary bypass; PDA^xx patent ductus arteriosus; ALCARPA° anomalous origin of the left coronary artery from the right pulmonary artery; RS to LCA°° right subclavian artery graft to left coronary artery; ACBG^a aorto-coronary bypass grafting; TPLSCA^aa transpulmonary artery subclavian artery graft to left coronary artery

only one graft was occluded and one was stenotic. Preoperative and postoperative comparisons frequently demonstrated growth of the vessel and the anastomosis.

Discussion

The subclavian artery, whether used in situ or as a free graft, provides excellent myocardial revascularization for ALCAPA results. Ligation of the left main coronary artery in ALCAPA is not an option. The myocardium remains ischemic, and the operative mortality rate for infants (less than 18 months of age) approaches 100%.[23] Aortocoronary artery vein grafts have been used with short-term success to correct ALCAPA,[18–20] but CPB is needed, and vein grafts do not enlarge as the patient grows.[21] El-Said et al.[24] have even documented stenotic lesions in vein grafts 2 to 5 years postsurgery. This conduit, then, is not as acceptable as the subclavian artery.

The IMA may be an alternative conduit used for myocardial revascularization in the pediatric age group 5 to 13 years old. The combination of bilateral IMA grafting with SV grafting was successfully used by Kitamura et al.[23] in children with Kawasaki disease. In 12 patients (11 boys, 1 girl), 17 IMA grafts and 11 SV grafts were constructed. Patency rates of the IMA grafts and SV grafts were 100% and 91%, respectively, in the early postoperative period (P = (not significant (NS)) and 100% and 50%, respectively, in a later follow-up period of greater than 1 year ($P < 0.05$). The in situ IMA graft was observed to enlarge 135% in length and 149% in diameter as the body surface area increased 112% ($P < 0.001$). The growth potential of both the IMA and the subclavian artery, which is not seen in the SV graft, is an important and unique characteristic to consider when revascularization of the myocardium is required in the pediatric age group. In conclusion, the right or left subclavian arteries are the choice conduits for the very young patient (less than 18 months), but either the IMA or subclavian artery are excellent alternative conduits for the older pediatric patient.

References

1. Apley J, Horton RE, Wilson MG. The possible role of surgery in the treatment of anomalous left coronary artery. Thorax 1957; 12:28–33.
2. Myer BW, Stefanik G, Stiles QR, Lindesmith GC, et al. A method of definitive surgical treatment of anomalous origin of left coronary artery: a case report. J Thorac Cardiovasc Surg 1968; 56:105–107.
3. Pinsky WW, Fagan LR, Kroeger RR, Mudd JFG, et al. Anomalous left coronary artery: report of two cases. J Thorac Cardiovasc Surg 1973; 65:810–814.
4. Horiuchi T, Suzuku Y, Iskizawa E. Successful subclavian-left coronary artery anastomosis for anomalous origin of left coronary in infancy. Tohoku J Exp Med 1975; 116:183–189.
5. Senderoff E, Slovis SJ, Moallem A, Kahn RE. Subclavian- coronary artery anastomosis: a technique for definitive correction of anomalous origin of left coronary artery. J Thorac Cardiovasc Surg 1976; 71:142–146.
6. Monro JL, Sharrott GP, Conway N. Correction of anomalous origin of left coronary artery using left subclavian artery. Br Heart J 1978; 40:79–82.
7. Yoshida Y, Emmanouilides GC, Nelsen RJ, Baylen BG, et al. Anomalous origin of the left coronary artery from the pulmonary artery: a case report with remarkable improvement of myocardial function following

subclavian artery-coronary artery anastomosis. Catheterization Cardiovasc Diagn 1980; 6:293–303.

8. Champsaur G, Bozio A, Joffre B, Brule P, et al. Anomalous origin of the left coronary artery from the pulmonary artery: treatment by left subclavian-left main coronary artery anastomosis. Nouv Presse Med 1980; 9(16):1167–1169.

9. Montigny M, Stanley P, Chartrand C, Selman E, et al. Postoperative evaluation after end to end subclavian-left coronary artery anastomosis in anomalous left coronary artery. J Thorac Cardiovasc Surg 1990; 100:270–273.

10. Neches WH, Mathews RA, Park SC, Lenox CC, et al. Anomalous origin of the left coronary artery from the pulmonary artery: a new method of surgical repair. Circulation 1974; 50:582–587.

11. Arciniegas E, Farooki ZQ, Hakimi M, Green EW. Management of anomalous left coronary artery from the pulmonary artery. Circulation 1980; 2(suppl. I)181–189.

12. Sanderson CJ, Anagnostopoulos CE, Brunner MC, Goluch L, et al. Growth in coronary-subclavian anastomosis: long-term clinical confirmation after treatment of anomalous left main coronary artery. J Thorac Cardiovasc Surg 1981; 82:293–296.

13. Laborde F, Marchand M, Leca F, Jarreau MM, et al. Surgical treatment of anomalous origin of the left coronary artery in infancy and childhood: early and late results in 20 consecutive cases. J Thorac Cardiovasc Surg 1981; 82:423–428.

14. Backer CL, Stout MJ, Vincent RZ, Muster AJ, et al. Anomalous origin of the left coronary artery: a twenty-year review of surgical management. J Thorac Cardiovasc Surg 1992; 103:1049–1058.

15. Takeuchi S, Imamura H, Katsumoto K, Hayashi I, et al. New surgical method for repair of anomalous left coronary artery from the pulmonary artery. J Thorac Cardiovasc Surg 1979; 78:7–11.

16. Doty DB, Chandramouli B, Schieken RE, Lauer RM, et al. Anomalous origin of the left coronary artery from the right pulmonary artery: surgical repair in a 10-month-old child. J Thorac Cardiovasc Surg 1976; 71:787–791.

17. Suzuki Y, Horiuchi T, Ishizawa E, Sato T, et al. Subclavian-coronary artery anastomosis in infancy for the Bland-White-Garland syndrome: a two year angiographic follow-up. Ann Thorac Surg 1978; 25:377–381.

18. Rowe GG, Young WP. Anomalous origin of the coronary arteries with special reference to surgical treatment. J Thorac Cardiovasc Surg 1960; 39:777–779.

19. Likar I, Criley JM, Lewis KB. Anomalous left coronary artery arising from the pulmonary artery in an adult: a review of the therapeutic problem. Circulation 1966; 33:727–732.

20. Cooley DA, Hallman GL, Bloodwell RD. Definitive surgical treatment of anomalous origin of the left coronary artery from pulmonary artery: indications and results. J Thorac Cardiovasc Surg 1966; 52:798–808.

21. Somerville J, Ross DN. Left coronary artery from the pulmonary artery: physiological considerations of surgical correction. Thorax 1970; 25:207–212.

22. Endo M, Takayasu S, Obunai Y, Nakazawa M, et al. Anomalous origin of left coronary artery from pulmonary artery: significance of saphenous vein bypass between aorta and left coronary artery. J Thorac Cardiovasc Surg 1974; 67:896–902.
23. Kitamura S, Seki T, Kawachi K, Moreta R, et al. Excellent patency and growth potential of internal mammary artery grafts in pediatric coronary artery bypass surgery. Circulation 1988; 70(suppl. I):129–139.
24. El-Said GM, Ruzyllo W, Williams RL, Mullins CE, et al. Early and late results of saphenous vein graft for anomalous origin of left coronary artery from pulmonary artery. Circulation 1973; 47–48(suppl. III):2–6.

11

The Lateral Costal Artery

Ronald K. Grooters and Hiroshi Nishida

The lateral costal artery (LCA), a common anomaly found present in 31 (27.6%) out of 112 cadavers studied by Kropp,[1] has been recently used for myocardial revascularization.[2] When present, about half of these arteries reach the fifth or sixth intercostal spaces.[1] If further study demonstrates this finding, it is likely that 10 to 15% of patients have the artery available to be used as a coronary bypass graft. This may, in part, have already been confirmed by Baurer et al.,[3] (Chapter 1) who demonstrated angiographically that large side branches were present in the internal mammary artery (IMA) 9% of the time. In the case report by Hartman et al.,[2] histological examination of the LCA and the IMA also demonstrated a close similarity. This evidence suggests that the LCA, like the IMA, may be resistant to atherosclerosis. It may make sense then for the surgeon to identify the presence of this conduit and use it as an alternative to the saphenous vein (SV) to enhance long-term outcomes in bypass patients.

Anatomy

In the study by Kropp,[1] all 112 cadavers were white; 104 were males and 8 were females. The artery was present in 31 (27.6%) subjects. It was more common on the left side. When it was present bilaterally, its length was not always the same.

The LCA usually arises just distal to the origin of the IMA (Fig. 1). It may also come from the subclavian or a high intercostal artery.

From Grooters RK and Nishida H: (editors): *Alternative Bypass Conduits and Methods for Surgical Coronary Revascularization.* © Futura Publishing Co., Inc., Armonk, NY, 1994.

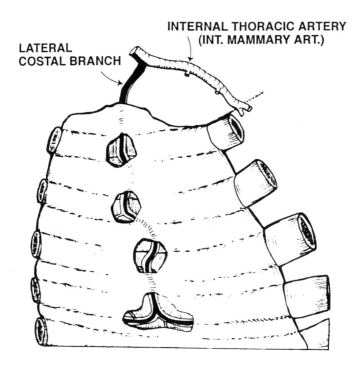

Fig. 1. Relationship of lateral costal artery (LCA) to the internal mammary artery (IMA) and chest wall. (Reprinted with permission from Grant JCB, Grant's Atlas of Anatomy, 6th ed., 1972, The Williams and Wilkins Company, Baltimore, Md.)

Then the artery courses along the midaxillary line or may be anterior to it. If this artery traverses six intercostal spaces, the caliber will be as large as the IMA.[4] Usually this artery is accompanied by two veins that drain into the subclavian vein. This artery also has branches, both anteriorly and posteriorly, which connect with each intercostal artery as it courses over the intercostal spaces.

Case Report

Hartman and colleagues[2] first described the utilization of this artery in bypassing a diagonal coronary artery. The patient with two-vessel coronary artery disease underwent a bilateral IMA revascularization. During the harvest of the left IMA, a large LCA was found originating from the proximal left IMA. An artery on the right side was also found. The left LCA was harvested as a pedicle including fascia and veins. The outer diameter was 2 mm, and the free flow measured 100 mL/min after a papaverine infusion into the artery. The length was 20 cm. This artery was then used to bypass a diagonal branch by constructing the anastomoses with 8-0 Prolene (Ethicon, Somerville, NJ). The right IMA was used to revascularize the right coronary artery (RCA), and the left IMA was used to bypass the left anterior descending (LAD). Repeat coronary catheterization demonstrated the left LCA to be patent.

Technique of Harvest

Hartman et al.[2] reported that this artery is easily seen after the chest wall is retracted. Reducing lung tidal volume by increasing the rate of ventilation augments the exposure. The artery is dissected from the chest wall using a method similar to that of harvesting the IMA in which a broad pedicle containing muscle, fascia, and veins together with the artery is created. The electrocautery blade is used to separate the pedicle from the ribs and intercostal muscles. Large branches from the pedicle were identified at each interspace and ligated with hemoclips. The harvest is continued proximal to the artery's junction with the IMA to gain complete mobility of the pedicle. A retrograde papaverine injection is done to achieve maximal arterial dilatation.

Discussion

The discovery that the LCA will occasionally be available as a conduit in a certain number of patients and that it histologically resembles the IMA will provide a challenge for surgeons to find the appropriate place for this artery. Many times, no doubt, we have ligated, ignored, or never identified this conduit, but now with the trend toward complete myocardial revascularization using arterial conduits, its utilization cannot be overlooked. Angiographic appearance, larger studies of this conduit's occurrence in the population, long-term follow-up, and further technical experience will determine the feasibility of this conduit. Once this information is known, the LCA may not be just an alternative, but as Hartman and colleagues[2] suggest, it can be viewed as an accessory IMA to be used.

References

1. Kropp BN. The lateral costal branch of the internal mammary artery. J Thorac Cardiovasc Surg 1951; 21:421–425.
2. Hartman AR, Mawulawde KI, Dervan JP, Anagnostopoulos CE. Myocardial revascularization with the lateral costal artery. Ann Thorac Surg 1990; 49:816–818.
3. Bauer EP, Bino MC, von Segesser AL, Turina MI. Internal mammary artery anomalies. Thorac Cardiovasc Surg 1990; 38:312– 315.
4. Adachi B. Das Arteriensystem der Japaner, Band 1. Kyoto, Japan, 1928:440.

Part IV
Alternative Bypass Methods Using the Internal Mammary Artery

12

Bilateral Internal Mammary Artery Usage

Ronald K. Grooters and Hiroshi Nishida

Simultaneous bilateral internal mammary artery (IMA) grafting is extensively used[1-3] and should be considered an attractive alternative method for a large percentage of patients requiring multivessel coronary artery revascularization. Barner[4] began using bilateral IMA grafting in 1972. Ten years later, both Barner et al.[5,6] and Bourassa et al.[7] produced angiographic evidence that atherosclerotic change in these arterial conduits was minimal. As discussed in Chapter 1, these conduits were shown to have better early patency rates[8] when compared to saphenous veins (SVs). The long-term patency rate for the IMA graft between 5 and 12 years postoperatively was definitely superior to the SV, 90% versus 50%, respectively.[8,9] Immunity of the IMA from atherosclerosis as a bypass conduit in the coronary position[10] and the angiographic observation that this graft can increase in size as dictated by myocardial blood demand[11] help establish a logic that using both IMAs for a myocardial revascularization procedure will be better for the patient than one IMA with venous conduits. Also, from our own observations of the literature and clinical experience, we feel that a rationale can be developed to provide answers to the questions of how and when it is best to use bilateral IMA grafting as an alternative that will enhance short- and long-term outcomes.

From Grooters RK and Nishida H: (editors): *Alternative Bypass Conduits and Methods for Surgical Coronary Revascularization.* © Futura Publishing Co., Inc., Armonk, NY, 1994.

Operative Techniques

Both IMAs are exposed through a standard median sternotomy incision using a modified Favoloro or Pittman retractor or a retractor of the surgeon's preference to expose the underside of the sternum and adjacent structures. Similar to the way Sewell described,[12] we use low-voltage electrocautery to divide fascia and muscle 1 cm on each side of the IMA. Care must be taken to avoid thermal damage to the artery and, proximally, to the phrenic nerve. The IMA is freed beyond the distal bifurcation. It is also appropriate to isolate the artery from the adjoining vein and fascia, particularly if the need for additional length for the graft is anticipated. After heparin is given, the grafts are divided distally and wrapped in a sponge wetted with a solution of papaverine (50 mg/50 mL of saline).

The free flow of each graft is assessed before the institution of cardiopulmonary bypass (CPB). We like to see flows greater than 90 cc/min if the graft is to be used for a large coronary artery and at least 120 cc/min if a sequential technique is anticipated. Flow rates of less than 50 cc/min reflect a conduit that is either small, obstructed, or damaged. This conduit may be used with a minor vessel, divided as a free graft to be used as a segment, or may have to be discarded. If the conduit is planned as a free graft, it is generally not divided proximally until just before it is used. This keeps it filled with blood and prevents possible ischemic damage.

The left IMA is most frequently considered to bypass the left anterior descending artery (LAD) and its branches or a large vessel from the circumflex artery (CX) such as the obtuse marginal. The in situ right IMA can be used to bypass a proximal CX via the transverse sinus, an LAD or its diagonal branches, a right coronary artery (RCA), or preferably, if long enough, the posterior descending artery, either routing it anterior or posterior to the inferior vena cava (Fig. 1). If the right IMA is planned as a free graft, the proximal anastomoses can be constructed with a running 6-0 or 7-0 polypropylene suture to the ascending aorta with its various options (Chapter 14, Fig. 1) or to the proximal left IMA as a Y graft (Fig. 2). If the left IMA is used as the site for proximal anastomosis, it is done prior to CPB so free-flow measurement of the free right IMA conduit is possible. By bringing the left IMA into better view from under the sternum and rotating its posterior surface anteriorly, suturing and placing the free graft onto the larger-diameter proximal left IMA is made easier. Bringing the free right IMA from the posterior aspect of the left IMA prevents

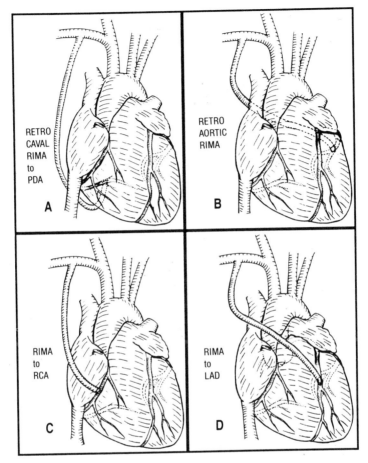

Fig. 1. Pathways used for the in situ right IMA. A— posterior to the inferior vena cava; B—retroaortic route through the transverse sinus; C—right lateral route to RCA; D— anterior route to LAD. Abbreviation: RIMA—right internal mammary artery.

twisting the left IMA, which may occur if the free right IMA originates from the anterior surface of the left IMA.

Before CPB is instituted, the grafts can frequently be estimated for appropriate length and point of placement on the coronary arteries. Dividing the pericardial sac anterior to the superior vena cava can sometimes allow better direct access to the transverse sinus or to

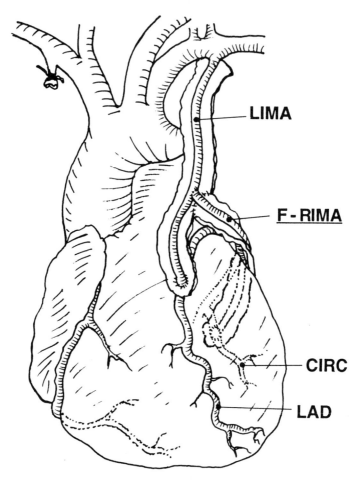

Fig. 2. Left IMA Y graft with RIMA free graft. (Reprinted with permission from Ann Thorac Surg 1990; 49:1015. Elsevier Science Publishing Co., New York, NY.)

a distal target on the RCA or its branches if the right IMA is used as an in situ graft. We also divide the left pleura and pericardium, as necessary, to provide a direct pathway for the in situ left IMA as it traverses beneath the apex of the left lung and anterior to the left hilum. This will keep the graft away from the sternum, assure adequate length, and prevent tension. Coronary anastomosis is performed with a continuous suturing technique using 7-0 or 8-0 polypropylene. Magnification (2.5–4.0 power) is used. Hypothermic

CPB (30°–32°C) and crystalloid or blood cardioplegia (4°–5°C) are used to keep septal myocardia temperatures between 10°–15°C. Aortic root venting is also a routine procedure.

Published Data

Operative Mortality

Barner et al.[5] were the first to report on bilateral IMA usage with an operative mortality rate of 8% (8 out of 100 patients). Anoxic arrest was used, and four of the deaths were from ventricular failure. Geha,[13] in 1976, had no mortality in 36 patients. In 1983, Lytle and colleagues[14] reported no deaths in 76 patients, but then, in 1986[15] after reviewing 500 patients, reported an operative mortality rate of 1.6% for the first 125 patients done between 1971 and 1982 and an operative mortality rate of 1.3% in the following 375 patients done between 1982 and 1984. Cameron et al.[16] also had no operative deaths in 36 patients reported in 1985, but Galbut et al.[17] recorded 9 deaths in 227 patients (4%). Cosgrove and his colleagues[2] in 1988 compared operative mortalities for vein-only usage, single IMA usage, and bilateral IMA usage. Each group had 338 patients, and the operative mortality rates were 6 (1.8%), 1 (0.3%), and 3 (0.9%), respectively. Kouchoukos et al.[3] showed no difference in 30-day mortality rates between single IMA grafting (2.8%) and bilateral IMA grafting (2.7%), but with vein-only procedures the rate was significant at 7.9% ($P = 0.001$). The largest study of bilateral IMA usage (1,087 patients) is reported by Galbut et al.[1] in 1990, with operative deaths in 29 patients (2.7%). The hospital mortality differed significantly with stable and unstable patients, 1.2% versus 5.3%, ($P < 0.005$). The presence of left main coronary artery disease or poor left-ventricular function did not make a significant difference.

Survival Rates

In the 1974 report by Barner,[4] the first-year survival rate for bilateral IMA grafting was 90%. By 1985, Galbut et al.[17] demonstrated a 99% survival rate at 1 year and in 1990,[1] after reviewing 1,087 patients with bilateral IMA usage, the one-year actuarial survival rate remained an excellent 98%. By 1983, Lytle and associates[14] reviewed 76 patients and reported an actuarial survival rate of 97.2% at 7 years and 90.2% at 9 years. Ten-year actuarial survival rates reported by

Galbut et al.[17,1] were 83% in 68 patients (1985) and 80% in a follow-up of 1,087 patients (1990). Fiore[18] reported similar ten-year survival rates at 84% and 82%, respectively, for 100 patients in a bilateral IMA group compared to 100 patients in the single IMA group. At 13 years, the survival rate was better for the bilateral IMA group (74%) versus the single IMA group (59%). In 1986, Cameron et al.[16] (Fig. 3) recorded cumulative survival rates in 748 coronary-bypass patients over the course of 15 years. Fourteen-year survival rates were 72% for single IMAs and 86% for bilateral IMAs, versus a 57% rate in the vein graft-only group, a significant difference ($P < 0.1$). Age-related survival rates at 15 years postoperatively from a review of 6,181 patients by Johnson et al. in 1989[19] for bilateral IMA usage demonstrated a 60% survival rate for patients age 50 or less at the time of operation and a 70% survival rate when the operation was done between the ages 50 and 60, but only a 44% rate of survival if the age at operation was between 60 and 70 years. (Chapter 1, Table 1). Most recently, Galbut et al.,[1] in 1990, has demonstrated a ten-year survival rate of 80% for patients receiving bilateral IMA grafts, which dropped to 56% at 17 years from the date of surgery.

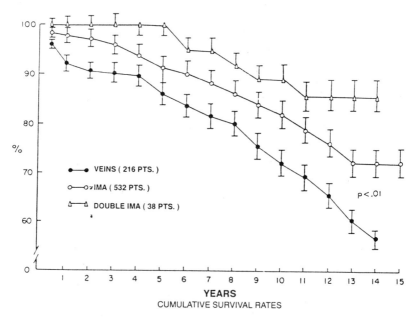

Fig. 3. Cumulative survival rates over 15 years (from Cameron A, et al.[16]).

Patency Rates

Postoperative catheterization revealed 80 out of 84 (95%) patent right IMA grafts and 82 out of 84 (97%) patent left IMA grafts in the Barner[4] report. In a follow-up at 1 year, patency rates were 22 out of 23 for right IMA grafts and 22 out of 22 for left IMA grafts. Eleven of 12 free grafts used were patent at the time of the postoperative angiography. All crossover right IMA grafts performed in 36 patients by Geha[13] in 1976 were angiographically visualized. Later (6 months to 2 years), a study of 10 patients revealed all right IMA grafts to be patent. Then, in 1983, Lytle and associates[14] demonstrated patency in 31 out of 35 (88.6%) in situ right IMA grafts and 18 out of 20 (90%) patent free IMA grafts at a mean postoperative interval of 26 months. Five years later, eight out of eight (100%) free grafts studied were patent. Puig et al.[20] studied postoperatively 17 retroaortic in situ right IMA grafts to the CX, and all were patent. In 1985, Galbut et al.[17] reported patency rates at a mean of 4½ years for both left IMA and right IMA grafts as 34 out of 37 (92%) and 26 of out 30 (87%), respectively. Patency rates of IMA grafts to specific coronary arteries ranged from 66.6% to 100% (Table 1). As of 1990, Fiore and colleagues[18] had reported a 13-year patency rate of 82% for left IMA grafts and 85% for right IMA grafts.

Rankin and colleagues[21] have suggested that problems can occur with the right IMA-circumflex marginal artery grafts brought through the transverse sinus. Two out of 20 grafts studied angiographically 1 to 32 weeks after operation were occluded, and 3 more exhibited slow flow. They discontinued this method and favored free IMA grafting techniques because of 100% patency (15 out of 15 patients). Loop et al.[22] specifically studied 40 free IMA grafts in the aortocoronary position within 18 months of surgery and found that 31 of 40 (77%) were patent. Technical problems with the aortic anastomosis were thought to be the cause of the increased closure rate. With grafts done later in the study, the patency rate improved to 91%.

Recurrence of Angina

Only 3 out of 100 patients developed recurrent angina at 1 year postoperatively in the first report (1974) by Barner.[4] Geha[13] noted recurrent angina in 17% of 36 patients within 2 years of bilateral IMA grafting. Clinical improvement was still present in 35 of 36 patients

Table 1
Postoperative Arteriography of Bilateral Internal Mammary Grafts in 53 Patients at a Mean Interval of 53.0 Months

Graft Site	Number of Grafts	Number Patent*
Left IMA		
LAD	31	28 (90.3)
DIAG/LAD	20	20 (100.0)
OM	11	10 (90.9)
DIAG	1	0 (0.0)
Total	63	58 (92.1)
Right IMA		
RCA/PDA	22	19 (86.3)
LAD	11	10 (90.9)
DIAG	3	2 (66.6)
OMB	17	14 (82.3)
Total	53	45 (84.9)

* Numbers in parenthesis are percentages.
IMA: internal mammary artery; DIAG: diagonal coronary artery; LAD: left anterior descending coronary artery; OM: obtuse marginal branch; PDA: posterior descending artery; RCA: right coronary artery
(From Galbut DL, et al.[1])

during the same time period. Lytle and associates[14] in a follow-up study at a mean interval of 67 months found 22 of 71 patients (31%) experiencing angina. The postoperative function was still improved in one New York Heart Association Class in 59 out of 71 patients (83%). Measuring symptom relief, Fiore et al.[18] in 1990 reported 100 patients with bilateral IMA grafting; 36% were asymptomatic at 13 years, versus 27% who were asymptomatic with single IMA grafting. Galbut et al.[1] also noted that, of 56 patients who followed a mean interval of 13.2 years, only 2 (3.5%) required reoperation. Of the remaining patients, 42 (75%) were asymptomatic, and 12 (21.4%) were NYHA Class II. In 1986, Cameron et al.,[16] who followed 38 patients, reported that recurrent angina was present in 21% of patients at 5 years, 30% at 10 years, and only 33% at 15 years.

Recurrence of Myocardial Infarction

In the report by Barner[4] in 1974, one patient developed a postoperative myocardial infarction (PMI). Among the 92 survivors at 1 year, Galbut and his group[17] in 1985 found that 12 out of 227 patients had experienced a nonfatal PMI during the follow-up period of 6 months to 12½ years. Cameron[16] in 1986 showed PMI rates of 7.8% within 5 years, 14% at 10 years, and 14% at 13 years in a follow-up of 36 patients. In the 1990 follow-up study by Galbut et al.,[1] 11 out of 56 patients (19%) developed PMI during a mean period of 13 years. Fiore et al.[18] compared 100 patients who had bilateral IMA grafting to 100 patients with a single IMA grafting plus vein grafts and demonstrated that 75% of the bilateral IMA group was free from PMI, versus 59% in the single IMA group.

Operative Morbidity

Perioperative Myocardial Infarction

Perioperative myocardial infarction rates are varied. The 1974 reports by Barner[4] quoted a rate of 4% in 100 patients, whereas Geha,[13] in 1976, had one perioperative infarction (2.7%) in 36 patients. Lytle[14] diagnosed the complication, defined as new electrocardiographic Q waves, in 6 out of 76 patients (7.9%) operated on from 1971 to 1980. Their infarction rate dropped to 2.7% of 375 patients done from 1982 to 1984.[15] By 1988, Cosgrove and colleagues[2] reported no significant differences in perioperative infarction rates for bilateral IMA grafting (2.1%), for single IMA grafting (0.9%), or vein graft only (0.6%). Galbut et al.[1] reviewed 1,087 patients in 1990 and found 22 patients (2.0%) with a perioperative myocardial infarction during bilateral IMA grafting.

Postoperative Bleeding

Bleeding, requiring reoperation, was experienced by 12% of 100 patients in the 1974 report by Barner.[4] Geha[13] had two out of 36 patients who required reoperation. Lytle[14] reported an 11.8% bleeding incidence in 1983 but then in 1986 demonstrated a reduction in reoperation for bleeding to 5%.[15] The number of transfusions per patient in the early group of 125 patients was 6.5 units, but the number decreased to 1.3 units in the 375-patient group done from 1982 to 1984. Kouchoukos and associates[3] reported no significant difference in the reoperation rate for bleeding in the bilateral IMA group (13 out of 246 patients, 5.3%), versus the single IMA group (32 out of 687 patients, 4.7%). The transfusion requirements per patient were similar:

2.1 units for the bilateral IMA group and 2.5 units for the single IMA group. Galbut et al.,[1] in 1990, noted reoperation for bleeding in 19 out of 1,087 patients (1.7%).

Sternal Infections

Mediastinitis developed in 4 out of 100 patients (4%) in the 1974 series of Barner.[4] Geha[13] had one 36-year-old patient become infected (2.7%). In 1983, Lytle and colleagues[14] reported a major sternal infection in only 1 out of 76 (1.3%) patients, and the rate remained low (8 out of 500 patients, 1.6%) in their 1986 report.[15] Patients with diabetes had an incidence of 4% (4 out of 98) in the same review. Kouchoukos et al.[3] reviewed 246 patients with bilateral IMA usage of which 6.9% became infected, versus 1.3% of 687 patients when one IMA was used. Diabetes and obesity were the major predictors in this series. A sternal infection developed in 19 out of 1,087 (1.7%) patients reviewed by Galbut et al.[1] in 1990. This report also noted that diabetes was a significant risk factor. In 1991, Grossi et al.[23] reported an 11.5% incidence (3 out of 26) among patients with diabetes and bilateral IMA grafting compared to a 3.8% incidence (5 out of 130 patients) in patients with bilateral IMA usage but without diabetes.

Discussion

Without question, most patients benefit from at least one IMA grafting (usually to the LAD) when multiple vessels need revascularization,[24] but does the second IMA graft provide additional benefit or increased risk? And, if so, when and how?

Various authors[1,2,18] have shown operative mortality rates using bilateral IMA grafting to be no different from single IMA or vein-graft-only usage. This most likely is a result of better anesthesia, improved myocardial preservation techniques, and more experience constructing the IMA-coronary anastomoses. In fact, poor ventricular function and left main disease are no longer risk factors. Unstable patients show a higher mortality rate than stable patients, 5.3% versus 1.2%, but no higher than when single IMA or vein-only techniques are used.[1] Operative mortality should not be a reason to withhold a bilateral IMA procedure.

Survival rates, both short term (1 year or less) and long term (greater than 5 years) are improved if at least one IMA is used.[14,16]

Even at 10 years, accumulated survival rates comparing one IMA used to bilateral IMA grafting (84% versus 82%) are excellent. At 13 years, postoperatively, the survival rates start to look better for the bilateral IMA group (74% versus 59%).[18] Cameron et al.,[16] in a small patient study, demonstrates better survival rates at 14 years with bilateral IMA usage (87%) than with single IMA grafting (72%). Johnson et al.[19] has additionally demonstrated that patient age at operation may be a predictor of survival rates when bilateral IMAs are used. If the patient is between 50 and 60 years old, the 15-year survival rate is the highest (70%). These data suggest that beyond 10 years postoperatively, bilateral IMA grafting may start to have more influence on survival, and the 50-to-60-year-old age group benefits the most.

Bilateral IMA myocardial revascularization is reported to be effective in relieving symptoms. Lytle and colleagues[14] have reported 69% of patients asymptomatic and 83% improved at a mean follow-up of 5 years postoperatively compared to their preoperative status. Fiore et al.[18] has shown that 36% of patients receiving bilateral IMA operations remain asymptomatic, whereas only 27% of patients receiving one IMA graft along with SV grafts remain without symptoms 13 years after surgery. Freedom from myocardial infarctions 17 years after surgery is also lower in the bilateral group (75%) than in the single IMA/SV group (59%). The relative immunity of these native IMA grafts to atherosclerotic changes seems to contribute to these long-term benefits.[25] Coupled with the characteristic that the IMA graft increases in size as coronary blood flow is demanded, bilateral IMA usage is extremely attractive, yet may be no better than a single IMA grafting with venous grafting until all myocardial events are studied for the postoperative period beyond 10 years.

Postoperative complications with bilateral IMA grafting were initially a concern. Additional dissection needed to harvest both arteries may have contributed to increased bleeding and transfusion usage, but with more experience, this may not be as much of a problem.[1] Increased operative and anesthesia time for harvesting both IMA grafts at first was thought to increase the possibility of intraoperative myocardial ischemia, but perioperative infarction rates (new onset Q waves) continued to remain low at 2%.[2,26] Mediastinitis is more frequent and as high as 6.9%,[3] but if bilateral IMA grafting is avoided in the obese diabetic patient,[1,14,23] this terrible and costly complication can be kept below a 2% rate.[1,15]

The Free Right IMA Graft and In Situ Left IMA Alternative

Crossover grafting of the right IMA in situ graft remains a concern. Reoperation can be very treacherous if this graft is patent and lies beneath the sternum. Using the in situ graft in a retroaortic manner can avoid this predicament, but it may then be too short to be used for extremely important vessels supplying a large amount of myocardium or for multiple anastomoses. The free right IMA graft can avoid the hazardous reoperation situation and, additionally, provide more length and opportunity for multiple sequential bypass techniques to reach the otherwise inaccessible distal posterior descending or CXs. An additional advantage is that this free grafting technique can provide a graft long enough to extend beyond diseased proximal coronary artery segments and onto the distal coronary that is without atherosclerosis. This is very important for a better long-term patency and fewer cardiac events. If the distal IMA diameter of an in situ graft does not have an adequate lumen (less than 1.5 mm), the poor distal segment can be removed if the IMA can be planned as a free graft, or it might otherwise be discarded. This free graft segment could then be used as part of a composite graft (see Chapter 15). Occasionally, the proximal portion of an IMA can be injured, or a subclavian artery stenosis is present. In those situations, again, the free graft technique may still be applicable.

The increased amount of operative time to harvest the additional IMA and the construction of the proximal anastomosis for the free graft IMA can be construed as disadvantageous. Also, the loss of an arterial conduit as a reserve for the future can later be detrimental to the patient when a redo operation is needed, but none of these reasons should entirely inhibit the consideration of bilateral IMA grafting. If the ideal patient for bilateral IMA grafting (the right IMA free graft with the in situ left IMA graft) can be identified, the surgeon may not have to revisit that patient's mediastinum as soon. So which patient might that be? We feel that a patient between the ages of 50 and 60 years (but not exclusively) with very significant double- or triple-vessel disease but without diffuse distal coronary artery pathology in whom most or all of the myocardium can be revascularized with this technique is the ideal candidate. If an operation is needed later in life, the crossover problem seen with the in situ right IMA graft will not be present.

In conclusion, significant short- and long-term additional benefits are present with bilateral IMA grafting. Using the additional right IMA as a free graft with the left IMA in situ can provide additional benefits in selected patients and is an attractive alternative to bilateral IMA in situ grafting or single IMA grafting with venous conduits.

References

1. Galbut DL, Traad EA, Dorman MJ, DeWitt PL, et al. Seventeen-year experience with bilateral internal mammary artery grafts. Ann Thorac Surg 1990; 49:195–201.
2. Cosgrove DM, Lytle BW, Loop FD, Taylor PC, et al. Does bilateral internal mammary artery grafting increase surgical risk. J Thorac Cardiovasc Surg 1988; 95:850–856.
3. Kouchoukos NT, Wareing TH, Murphy SF, Pilate C, et al. Risks of bilateral internal mammary artery bypass grafting. Ann Thorac Surg 1990; 49:210–219.
4. Barner HB. Double internal mammary-coronary artery bypass. Arch Surg 1974; 109:627–630.
5. Barner HB, Swartz MT, Mudd JG, Tyros DH. Late patency of the internal mammary artery as a coronary bypass conduit. Ann Thorac Surg 1982; 34:408.
6. Barner HB, Standeven JW, Reese J. Twelve-year experience with internal mammary artery for coronary artery bypass. J Thorac Cardiovasc Surg 1985; 90:668–675.
7. Bourassa MG, Enjalbert M, Campeau L, Lesperance J. Progression of atherosclerosis in coronary arteries and bypass grafts: ten years later. Am J Cardiol 1984; 53:102C.
8. Grondin CM, Campeau L, Lesperance J, Enjalbert M, et al. Comparison of late changes in internal mammary and saphenous vein grafts in two consecutive series of patients 10 years after operation. Circulation 1984; 70(suppl. 1):208–212.
9. Lytle BW, Loop FD, Cosgrove DM, Ratcliff NB, et al. Long-term (5–12 years) serial studies of internal mammary artery and saphenous vein bypass grafts. J Thorac Cardiovasc Surg 1985; 89:248–258.
10. Tector AJ, Schmohl TM, Jansen B, Kallies PA-C, et al. The internal mammary artery graft: its longevity after coronary bypass. JAMA 1981; 246:2181–2183.
11. Singh RN, Big RA, Kay EB. Physiological adaptability: the secret of success of the internal mammary artery grafts. Ann Thorac Surg 1986; 41:247–250.
12. Sewell WH. Surgery for Acquired Coronary Artery Disease. Springfield, Ill.: Charles C. Thomas Publisher, 1967.
13. Geha AS. Cross double internal mammary-to-coronary-artery grafts. Arch Surg 1976; 111:289–292.

14. Lytle BW, Cosgrove DM, Saltus GL, Taylor PC, et al. Multivessel coronary revascularization without saphenous vein: long-term results of bilateral internal mammary artery grafting. Ann Thorac Surg 1983; 36(5):540–547.
15. Lytle BW, Cosgrove DM, Loop FD, Borsh J, et al. Perioperative risk of bilateral internal mammary artery grafting: analysis of 500 cases from 1971 to 1984. Circulation 1986; 74(suppl. III):37–41.
16. Cameron A, Kemp HG Jr, Green GE. Bypass surgery with the internal mammary graft: 15 year follow-up. Circulation 1986; 74(suppl. III):30–36.
17. Galbut DL, Traad EA, Dorman MJ, DeWitt PL, et al. Twelve-year experience with bilateral internal mammary artery grafts. Ann Thorac Surg 1985; 40(3):264–270.
18. Fiore AC, Nounhein KS, Dean P, Kaiser GC, et al. Results of internal thoracic artery grafting over 15 years: single versus double grafts. Ann Thorac Surg 1990; 49:202–209.
19. Johnson WD, Brenowitz JB, Kayser KL. Factors influencing long-term (10 years to 15 years) survival after successful coronary artery bypass operation. Ann Thorac Surg 1989; 48:19–25.
20. Puig LB, Neto LF, Rari M, Ramires JAF, et al. A technique of anastomosis of the right internal mammary artery to the circumflex artery and its branches. Ann Thorac Surg 1984; 38(5):533–534.
21. Rankin JS, Newman GE, Bashore TM, Muhlbaier LH, et al. Clinical and angiographic assessment of complex mammary artery bypass grafting. J Thorac Cardiovasc Surg 1986; 92:832–846.
22. Loop FD, Lytle BW, Cosgrove DM, Golding LAR, et al. Free (aorta-coronary) internal mammary artery graft: late results. J Thorac Cardiovasc Surg 1986; 92:927–931.
23. Grossi EA, Esposito R, Harris LJ, Crooke GA, et al. Sternal wound infections and use of internal mammary artery grafts. J Thorac Cardiovasc Surg 1991; 102:342–347.
24. Loop FD, Lytle BW, Cosgrove DM, et al. Influence of the internal mammary artery graft on 10-year survival and other cardiac events. N Engl J Med 1984; 314:1–6.
25. Singh RN, Sosa JA, Green GE. Long term fate of the internal mammary artery and saphenous vein grafts. J Thorac Cardiovasc Surg 1983; 86:359–363.
26. Tector AJ, Schmahl TM, Canino VR. Expanding the use of the internal mammary artery to improve patency in coronary artery bypass grafting. J Thorac Cardiovasc Surg 1986; 91:9–16.

13

Sequential Internal Mammary Artery Grafting

Ronald K. Grooters and Hiroshi Nishida

Expanding the usage of the internal mammary artery (IMA) graft by using sequential coronary artery grafting techniques is now a necessary alternative in the cardiac surgeon's armamentarium. In the 1970s, the vein graft and its use as a sequential graft developed into a routine,[1-4] and today it is still a useful technique that reaches vessels on the posterior and inferior surfaces of the heart and also preserves venous conduit. As reports of better short- and long-term patency rates with an IMA graft as compared to a venous graft became apparent in the early 1980s,[5-8] surgeons logically speculated and then demonstrated that grafting more coronary arteries with IMA conduits might enhance longevity and decrease adverse cardiac events following coronary artery bypass grafting. Although the extent to which sequential IMA grafting benefits a group of patients has not been determined, the mere fact that the IMA graft is resistant to atherosclerosis[9,10] compels the use of IMA sequential combinations.

An initial concern that since IMA graft flow was less than vein graft flow the IMA graft, therefore, was inadequate for sequential grafting has been dispelled by studies[11,12] showing that IMA graft flow increases with time and demand. Additionally, the flow reserve of sequential IMA grafts has been demonstrated to be equivalent to that found in nonstenotic native coronary arteries.[13] Another fear, that the increase in technical demand with IMA grafting would pro-

From Grooters RK and Nishida H: (editors): *Alternative Bypass Conduits and Methods for Surgical Coronary Revascularization.* © Futura Publishing Co., Inc., Armonk, NY, 1994.

125

duce more complications, such as postoperative bleeding, perioperative infarctions, and suboptimal symptom relief, has not been realized. Since Kabbani and colleagues[14] reported the initial usage of sequential IMA grafting, surgeons have gained experience with IMA grafting techniques, and along with improved myocardial preservation techniques, better long-term clinical results using the IMA sequential graft are reported without a significant increase in postoperative problems (Table 1). Grafting as many coronary arteries as is feasibly possible with an IMA conduit using sequential grafting methods does depend on anatomy, but sequential grafting has become a routine procedure of choice, whenever possible, for coronary revascularization. It is not just another alternative in cases in which there is inadequate conduit or an atherosclerotic ascending aorta as initially suggested by Kabbani and colleagues in 1983.[14]

Technique

After the median sternotomy incision is made, one or both of the IMAs are harvested using a technique similar to Sewell[15] or Mills.[16] A wide pedicle is created using low-voltage electrocautery, which includes the vein, muscle, fascia, and adipose tissue that surrounds the IMA. This method prevents injury during harvest and helps identify twisting the conduit during its use. Once the IMA pedicle is completed and mobilized from the level of the xiphoid distally to the area of the phrenic nerve and proximally to the subclavian vein, it is wrapped with papaverine-soaked sponges. There is a total divergence of technique among surgeons on how to handle the IMA at this point. Boustany and Mills[17] have described a technique of graft injection with a papaverine solution, diluted 1:40 in nonheparinized plasma-lyte A with a pH of 7.4 (Travenol Lab, Inc., Deerfield, Ill.), which assists in the dilatation of the graft and detection of side-branch leaks. Both Tector and his group[18] and Dion and colleagues,[19] on the other hand, do not routinely use papaverine or any other vasodilating agents on the IMA.

Once cannulation has taken place and before institution of cardiopulmonary bypass (CPB), the IMA is divided distally, and free flow is measured after the distal end of the graft is inspected and prepared. A minimum of 100 cc/min of flow is necessary for the sequential technique to be considered. If it is not obtained, the graft is considered for use as a free graft or a single coronary artery graft,

Table 1

Sequential Bypass Statistics by Author

Author/Date	No. of Pts.	Predominant Sequence/No. of Pts.	Operative Deaths No./%	Periop. Myoc. Infarc. No./%	Catheterization Results
Kabbani[14] 1983	8	Diag-LAD/6	0/0	0/0	4 patients; 100% patency (2–5 yrs)
McBride[25] 1983	39	Diag-LAD/37	0/0	1/37; (2.6)	10 patients; 100% patency (1 mo–5 yrs)
Harjola[20] 1984	61	Diag-LAD/59	++2/61; 3.3	NR	50 patients/98/101; 1,984 anast. patent; mean 35.1 mos
Kamath[22] 1985	87	Diag-LAD/45 Marg-Marg/22	0/0	2/67;+ (2.9)	84 sequential anastomoses; 93% patency (1 yr)
Hodgson[13] 1986	20	Diag-LAD/9	0/0	NR	1 graft occluded; 90% patency (time of study unknown)
Russo[26] 1986	45	Diag-LAD/38 LAD-LAD/2	1/190*; 0.5	4/190*; 2.1	108 sequential anast. 98.2% patent (time of study unknown)
Rankin[21] 1986	207	Diag-LAD/134 Marg to CX/15	NR	NR	133/134 grafts patent; 15/15 grafts patent 1–32 wks
Boustany[17] 1988	50	Diag-LAD/46 LAD to LAD/2	0/0 0/0	0/0 0/0	11 patients/0 closures or defects (time of study unknown)
Tector[18] 1989	543	Diag-LAD/516	17/718**; 2.4	NR	actuarial survival at 6 yrs— 92.5%
Dion[19] 1989	231	Diag-LAD/152 CX-CX-11	6/231; 2.6	12/231; 5.2	325/342 anast.; (95%) patent; 1 IMA graft closed at 6 mos

*: includes other IMA usage; **: rate includes bilateral IMA usage; +: technetium 99 m pyrophosphate scan; ++: deaths due to poor ventricular function preop; NR: not reported; Diag: diagonal; Marg: marginal; anast.: anastomoses

usually to the left anterior descending (LAD), or it is discarded if the flow is less than 50 cc/min as a result of injury or atherosclerosis. When possible, prior to CPB, the graft is laid over the surface of the heart to determine if the length is adequate for use in the diagonal-LAD sequence. The left pleura and the pericardium at the level of the left hilum may need dividing to provide a shorter, more direct route to the targeted vessels. CPB is then instituted. If the circumflex system is considered for sequential grafting, the IMA conduit can be measured, and the lie of the graft approximated at this time. If, after inspecting and estimating the graft's length and pathway relationship to the coronary vessels to be grafted, it is determined that sequential grafting may not be feasible, this technique is abandoned, and the IMA is grafted to the most important vessel (the LAD or a large obtuse marginal). The smaller, less important vessels are then considered for a place in a sequential venous conduit or any other available arterial conduit such as a free right IMA or gastroepiploic artery. We agree with Boustany and Mills[17] that if the lateral distance between the proposed diagonal and LAD is greater than 4 cm and the angle is more than 60° (Fig. 1), the sequential technique should be avoided and alternatives should be considered.

Side-to-Side Anastomosis

After cardioplegia has been given, the venous grafts, if any, are completed first. This lessens the amount of manipulation of the heart to which the IMA graft may otherwise be subjected. We then construct the side-to-side anastomosis first. After identifying the points on the IMA graft and the coronary artery for anastomotic placement, both are opened about 0.8–1.0 cm. The suturing, using 7-0 or 8-0 polypropylene, is started usually at the heel of the graft from the outside to the inside and then brought through the heel of the coronary artery incision from the inside to the outside, trying to pick up a small portion of epicardium to add strength to the suture line of the heel. Two or three passes of the suture are made (Fig. 2) before the graft and the coronary artery are approximated and the anastomosis is completed. This technique requires intermittent traction on the sutures and frequent inspection of the inside of the anastomosis to detect loose sutures (loops), intimal flaps, arterial tears, and inappropriate suture placement, such as catching the opposite wall of the artery or graft. Prior to finishing the anastomosis, the artery is probed both distally and proximally.

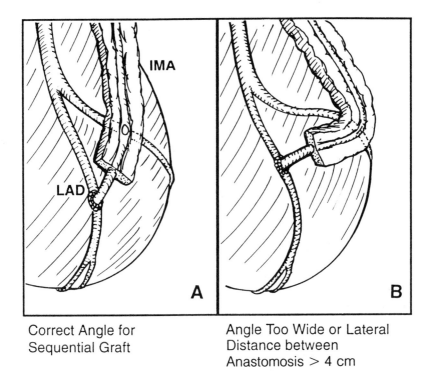

| Correct Angle for Sequential Graft | Angle Too Wide or Lateral Distance between Anastomosis > 4 cm |

Fig. 1. (A) The geometry of the left anterior descending (LAD) and diagonal branches is considered in planning a sequential anastomosis. When there is a small angle between the LAD and the diagonal branch, a sequential anastomosis between these two vessels is very feasible. (B) However, if the lateral distance between the proposed diagonal artery and the LAD is greater than 4 cm and their angle is more than about 60°, a sequential anastomosis is generally avoided. This is due to the tendency for kinking of the graft just proximal to the sequential anastomosis. (from Boustany CW Jr., et al.[17]).

We generally avoid the perpendicular side-to-side ("diamond") anastomosis, unless using this technique looks advantageous. This usually means that the IMA graft diameter is large (2–3 mm). We proceed cautiously by opening the first coronary artery of the sequential only a few millimeters (2 or 3 mm) to prevent the "seagull" deformity illustrated by Grondin and Limer[3] (Fig. 3). This anastomosis is always started on the side of the graft that will become the heel once the two vessels are approximated (Fig. 4a). It is then finished by suturing the side opposite the surgeon first, coming around the toe of the coro-

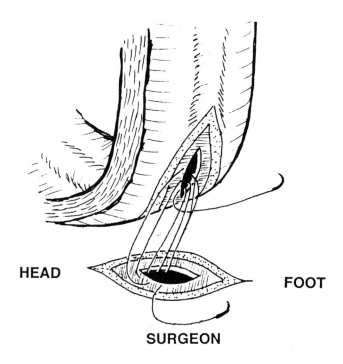

Fig. 2. Parallel side-to-side anastomosis begun with two or three passes of the suture prior to approximation of the graft and coronary artery (from Tector AJ, et al.[18]).

nary arteriotomy, opening it more at this point if needed, and then finishing the remaining side of the anastomosis. A continuous 8-0 polypropylene suturing technique is used to save time and assure a hemostatic "diamond" opening (Fig. 4b).

We then proceed to the distal end-to-side anastomosis after more cardioplegia is given. Construction of this graft is also started at the heel by placing two continuous sutures outside-in on the heel of the graft and then bringing the sutures inside-out at the matching heel of the coronary arteriotomy before lowering the graft to approximate the artery. This same continuous suturing technique can be used for this end-side anastomosis whether the IMA graft is parallel or perpendicular to the arteriotomy. We always try to develop a "cobrahead" configuration for this distal anastomosis. We occasionally

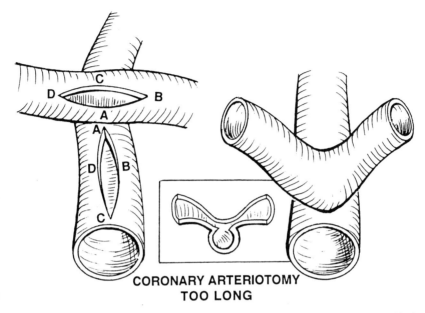

CORONARY ARTERIOTOMY
TOO LONG

Fig. 3. Short arteriotomies are mandatory in order to avoid a so-called "seagull" deformity (from Boustany CW Jr, et al.[17]).

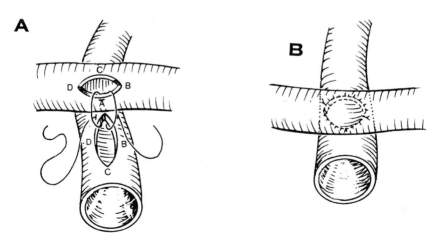

Fig. 4. Suturing is performed such that the angle of the coronary artery is sewn to the midwall of the IMA graft (A) and continued to B, C, and D. (B) The finished "diamond" anastomosis without narrowing (from Boustany CW Jr, et al.[17])

place the side-to-side anastomosis on the LAD and then bring the distal limb of the IMA graft over to the diagonal. This frequently necessitates the perpendicular end-to-side technique on the diagonal branch (Fig. 5) but assures the LAD the high blood flow of the larger proximal IMA graft. Once the anastomoses have been constructed, the vascular occlusion clamp is removed to identify bleeding points and correct them as necessary. The heel of the anastomosis is the most frequent site for bleeding. Also, if any hematomas develop in

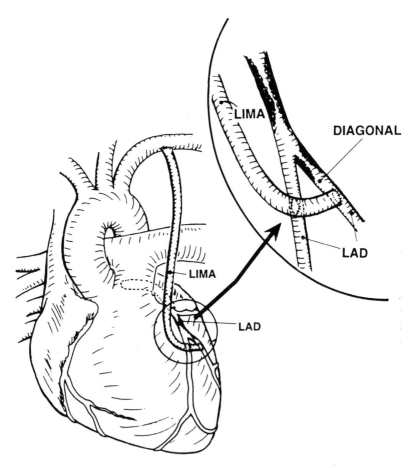

Fig. 5. Diagrammatic representation of sequential IMA grafting with the diagonal branch being the last to assure the LAD the maximum blood flow.

the adventitia or perivascular tissue at the graft sites, this tissue is opened with a pair of Potts scissors and the point of bleeding is corrected. Twisting and kinking, if present, need to be corrected, which usually means redoing the anastomosis. If the graft looks satisfactory, the pedicle tissue is tacked to the epicardium with 5-0 or 6-0 polypropylene sutures to prevent tension on the anastomosis. The cross-clamp is released, and the operation is finished, but if, near the completion of the surgery (once off CPB and ventilating), tension on the proximal segment of the graft is detected, consideration is then given to converting the in-situ IMA graft to a free graft and suturing the proximal anastomosis where convenient and safe (Chapter 14). This problem is more frequently seen if the right IMA is used in situ to the circumflex system.

Results

Operative Mortality

Sequential grafting does not seem to affect operative mortality rates, which range from 0%–3.3% (Table 1). The highest rates reported by Harjola et al.,[20] Tector et al.,[18] and Dion et al.[19] include patients with severe left ventricular dysfunction, elderly patients in their eighth and ninth decades, and patients needing emergency coronary artery bypass grafting for failed coronary angioplasty. We have also reviewed our latest 217 patients receiving at least one sequential grafting from 1990–1992, and we sustained only two deaths (< 1%). One patient died from a massive perioperative stroke, and the other, who preoperatively had an ejection fraction of 20% in addition to having a redo operation, died from low cardiac output. This has compared favorably to our overall operative mortality rate of 3.1% for patients not receiving a sequential graft over the same period.

Patency Rates

Patency rates studied postoperatively range from 90% to 100% (Table 1). These are results from angiography done at various time periods postoperatively. One of the most complete studies comparing patency rates of different sequential grafts is by Rankin and colleagues.[21] This group angiographically studied 207 patients from 1 to 32 weeks after operation and found patency rates of distal anastomoses to be 90% (196 out of 218) for sequential vein grafts, 99% (133 out of 134) for the IMA sequential graft to the LAD systems, 100% (15 out of 15) for the IMA sequential graft to the circumflex system, and 100% (6 out of 6) for the sequential IMA free graft. Dion's group[19] also studied a significant number of patients (157) an average of 6 months after operation (range: 5 to 13 months). Including vessels requiring an endarterectomy, 95% of the sequential IMA anastomoses were patent.

Symptom Relief

Kamath et al.[22] reported that 79 out of 83 patients during a mean follow-up period of 21 months were found to have complete symptom relief and 3 other patients had obtained considerable relief, although minimal angina symptoms remained. Exercise stress tests were performed on 64 patients. In this group, 54 patients had a negative test, 7 patients had an equivocal test, none had a positive test, and 3 patients were not available for testing. Kabbani and colleagues[14] reviewed their original eight patients with sequential IMA grafting and noted that all patients were angina free after operation for a follow-up period of up to 6 years.

Postoperative Bleeding

In our review of 217 patients with sequential grafting (1990–1992), only 3 patients (1.5%) needed a return trip to the operating room for postoperative bleeding. The bleeding site in one patient was from the heel of the distal anastomosis, coagulopathy was the cause of bleeding in another patient, and no cause for bleeding could be found in the third patient. Rankin and his colleagues[21] reported that only 7 out of 207 patients (3.3%) required a reoperation for bleeding. This group of patients included other complex mammary artery bypass grafting such as free grafting and bilateral IMA grafting.

Graft Flow Reserve Study

Hodgson and investigators[13] measured coronary flow reserve in various grafts after a contrast-induced hyperemia with an intragraft injection of 5 to 7 mL of Renografin-76 (E.R. Squibb & Sons, Princeton, NJ) by a digital subtraction angiographic technique. This was done an average of 25 days after surgery in 20 patients. The flow estimates for a given myocardial region were obtained by division of the vascular volume variable (intensity) by the time of appearance of contrast (cycles) for each myocardial region of interest. The coronary flow reserve was calculated as a ratio of flow estimate obtained during the hyperemia injection and the flow estimate obtained during the initial basal flow study. No difference was found in coronary flow reserve between the proximal and distal anastomotic regions in either the sequential IMA graft group 2.14 ± 0.50 versus 2.29 ± 0.68, n = 8, P = NS) or the sequential vein group (1.77 ± 0.49 versus 2.08 ± 0.78, n = 6, P = NS). The flow reserve of the sequential IMA graft was not different from that provided by a single IMA graft (1.64 ± 0.39, n = 5), a single vein graft (1.95 ± 0.95, n = 15), or a nonstenotic native coronary artery (2.04 ± 0.87, n = 34).

Discussion

Following the report by Kabbani et al.[14] describing the use of IMA sequential grafting as an alternative because of inadequate veins or an atherosclerotic ascending aorta, other surgeons[10,17,22,23] sought to evolve this technique for routine usage. The initial concern about the necessary meticulous nature of this method, requiring prolonged and possibly hazardous myocardial ischemic times, has been dispelled. No increase in perioperative myocardial infarction rates occurred (Table 1), of which the highest rates were 3.3% and 5.2%.[19,20] Adequate IMA flow is also present for most sequential graft situations, and flow reserve to meet increased demand has been documented.[11,12] This was also nicely demonstrated by Tector and his colleagues[24] on a patient requiring reoperation. At the initial surgery, the IMA graft flow measured only 20 mL/min and then, at reoperation 9 years later, the same IMA graft had a 90 mL/min flow rate. They concluded that if the IMA graft flow was enough to sustain adequate initial myocardial perfusion, it could also increase with time and demand. These findings added to the well-documented facts[9,10] that the IMA graft is very resistant to atherosclerosis and that patency rates of 90% at 10 years—in contrast to patency rates of 50% or less over the same time period for saphenous vein (SV) grafts—provide improved long-term clinical results[6-8] makes sequential IMA grafting a method of choice whenever possible.

Techniques may vary, but this doesn't seem to matter. Tector and his group[18] have used complex IMA grafting extensively; they do not routinely use papaverine or measure IMA graft flow but, nevertheless, have excellent results. Boustany and Mills[17] dilate the IMA with a unique papaverine injection to assist its dilatation and routine measure flow. They prefer to graft the LAD before proceeding to the sequence of the diagonal branch to assure a correct lie of the graft to the most important vessel (usually the LAD). Of the many surgeons who have reported on this technique (Table 1), all surely have their own special variations of this method, yet excellent patency rates and low complication rates are consistently reported.

A word of caution. There are many combinations for sequential grafting (Table 2) from Tector's report in 1984,[24] but he has recommended, and we concur, that two major coronary arteries (i.e., the LAD and circumflex (CX) coronary artery) generally should not be grafted with the same IMA conduit. Also, the surgeon must feel comfortable constructing the sequential graft on a particular patient. A nice rule-of-thumb that we still find useful in preventing flow problems was previously described by McBride and Barner[25]; the IMA should be equal to or greater in size than the larger of the two vessels to be grafted. If the surgeon also feels that (1) the patient's coronary anatomy is suitable, (2) the location and extent of atherosclerosis is not a problem, (3) the quality of the IMA graft is good (no atherosclerosis), (4) the method or origin (in situ or free) of the IMA graft is appropriate, and (5) the clinical condition of the patient is stable, he

---

Table 2
Possible Combinations of Left and Right Internal Mammary Artery (IMA) Sequential Grafts

Left IMA		Right IMA	
Side-to-Side	End-to-Side	Side-to-Side	End-to-Side
Diag	LAD	LAD	Diag
Diag-diag	LAD	Diag	Cx Marg
LAD	Diag	Cx Marg	Cx Marg
Diag	Cx Marg		
Cx Marg	Cx Marg		

Diag: diagonal branch; Cx Marg: marginal branch of the circumflex coronary artery
(From Tector AJ, et al.[24])

or she can then proceed with sequential grafting. If all of these considerations do not seem optimal, sequential IMA techniques should not be forced into the coronary bypass operation, and the surgeon should be ready to accept a single IMA graft and use alternative techniques or conduits. Lastly, the viability of the myocardial segment that receives the sequential graft is most important. It does the patient little good to construct a nice diagonal-LAD sequential IMA graft to a heart with a completed anterior wall infarct or scarring from a previous old injury. Always graft the IMA to coronary arteries that supply viable myocardium.

Measures to enhance IMA graft flow include careful dissection and meticulous preparation (including the use of papaverine in some way); the creation of nice "cobra-head" distal anastomosis without graft narrowing; placement of the proximal side-to-side anastomosis to the larger coronary artery; the use of either parallel or perpendicular anastomosis to keep the sequential segment as short as possible; and the use of an IMA (right or left) as a free graft. If all of these measures are given consideration, then sequential grafting will safely give the patient the maximum benefit the IMA has to offer.[26] Multiple IMA grafts, of which sequentialling is a part, should have a major impact on the long-term results of coronary bypass surgery. How and to what the sequential grafting is constructed constitutes the alternatives the surgeon has to decide upon for each patient.

References

1. Sewell WH, Sewell KV. Technique for the coronary snake graft operation. Ann Thorac Surg; 22:58–65.
2. Cheanvechi C, Groves LK, Surakiatchchanukul S, Tanaka H, et al. Bridge saphenous vein graft. J Thorac Cardiovasc Surg 1975; 70:63–68.
3. Grondin CM, Limer R. Sequential anastomoses in coronary artery grafting: technical aspects and early and late angiographic results. Ann Thorac Surg 1976; 23:1–8.
4. Moreno-Cabral RJ, Mamuja RG, Dang CR. Multiple coronary artery bypass using sequential technique. Am J Surg 1977; 134:64–69.
5. Grondin CM, Campeau L, Lesperance J, Enjalbert M, et al. Comparison of late changes in internal mammary artery and saphenous vein grafts in two consecutive series of patients 10 years after operation. Circulation 1984; 70(suppl. I):I208–I212.
6. Galbut DL, Traod EA, Dorman MJ, DeWitt PL, et al. Twelve-year experience with bilateral internal mammary artery grafts. Ann Thorac Surg 1985; 40(3):264–270.

7. Cameron A, Kemp HG JR, Green GE. Bypass surgery with the internal mammary artery graft: 15 year follow-up. Circulation 1985; 74(suppl. III):30–36.

8. Fiore AC, Nounhein KS, Dean P, Kaiser GC, et al. Results of internal thoracic artery grafting over 15 years: single versus double grafts. Ann Thorac Surg 1990; 48:202–209.

9. Sims RH. A comparison of coronary and internal mammary arteries and implications of the results in the etiology of arteriosclerosis. Am Heart J 1983; 105:560–566.

10. Tector AJ, Schmohl TM, Jansen B, Kallies PA-C, et al. The internal mammary artery graft: its longevity after coronary bypass. JAMA 1981; 246:2181–2183.

11. Singh RN, Big RA, Kay EB. Physiological adaptability: the secret of success of the internal mammary artery grafts. Ann Thorac Surg 1986; 41:247–250.

12. Vogel JHK, McFadden B, Spence R, Jahuke EJ Jr, et al. Quantitative assessment of myocardial performance and graft patency following coronary artery bypass with the internal mammary artery. J Thorac Cardiovasc Surg 1978; 75:487–498.

13. Hodgson JM, Singh AK, Drew TM, Riley RS, et al. Coronary flow reserve provided by sequential internal mammary artery grafts. J Am Coll Cardiol 1986; 7:32–37.

14. Kabbani SS, Hanna ES, Bashour TT, Crew JR, et al. Sequential internal mammary-coronary artery bypass. J Thorac Cardiovasc Surg 1983; 86:697–702.

15. Sewell WH. Surgery for acquired coronary artery disease. Springfield, Ill.: Charles C. Thomas, Publisher, 1967.

16. Mills NL. Physiologic and technical aspects of the internal mammary artery-coronary artery bypass grafts. In: Cohn LH, ed. Modern Technics in Cardiac Surgery/Thoracic Surgery, VII. Mount Kisco, N. Y.: Futura Publishing Co., 1980:48-1–48-19.

17. Boustany CW Jr, Mills NL. Sequential coronary artery bypass utilizing the internal mammary artery. J Cardiovasc Surg 1988; 29:123–127.

18. Tector AJ, Schmahl TM, Crouch JD, Canino VR, et al. Sequential, free and Y internal thoracic artery grafts. Eur Heart J 1989; 10(suppl. H): 71–77.

19. Dion R, Verhelst R, Rousseau M, Goenen M, et al. Sequential mammary grafting: clinical, functional, and angiographic assessment 6 months postoperatively in 231 consecutive patients. J Thorac Cardiovasc Surg 1989; 98:80–89.

20. Harjola PT, Frich MH, Jarjula A, Jarvinen A, et al. Sequential internal mammary artery (IMA) grafts in coronary artery bypass surgery. Thorac Cardiovasc Surg 1984; 32:288–292.

21. Rankin JS, Newman GE, Bashore TM, Muhlbaier LH, et al. Clinical and angiographic assessment of complex mammary artery bypass grafting. J Thorac Cardiovasc Surg 1986; 92:832–846.

22. Kamath ML, Matysik LS, Schmidt DH, Smith LL. Sequential internal mammary artery grafts. J Thorac Cardiovasc Surg 1985; 89:163–169.

23. Tector AJ, Schmahl TM, Canino VR. Expanding the use of the internal mammary artery to improve patency in coronary artery bypass grafting. J Thorac Cardiovasc Surg 1986; 91:9–16.
24. Tector AJ, Schmahl TM. Techniques for multiple internal mammary artery bypass grafts. Ann Thorac Surg 1984; 38:281–286.
25. McBride LR, Barner HB. The left internal mammary artery as a sequential graft to the left anterior descending system. J Thorac Cardiovasc Surg 1983; 86:703–705.
26. Russo P, Orazulok TA, Schaff HV, Holmes DR Jr. Use of internal mammary artery grafts for multiple coronary artery bypasses. Circulation 1986; 74(suppl. III):III-48–III-52.

14

The Internal Mammary Artery Free Graft

Ronald K. Grooters and Hiroshi Nishida

The first reported internal mammary artery (IMA) free graft used as a coronary artery bypass conduit was reported by Loop and colleagues[1] in 1972. This patient had severe stenotic lesions of both the anterior descending and the right coronary artery (RCA). The saphenous veins (SVs) had previously been stripped. The free IMA was successfully interposed between the aorta and the distal RCA. Angiography confirmed the graft to be patent. In 1973, this same group[2] studied the flow rates of free IMA grafts to coronary arteries in four patients. No important differences between free IMA and in situ IMA grafts were found. The IMA also remains resistant to atherosclerosis even as a free graft[3] to provide long-term patency, anginal relief, and survival. This provides the justification to use the free IMA conduit in a variety of methods during coronary artery revascularization.

Why and When to Use

At present, three conditions need to be kept in mind to provide justification for the use of a free IMA graft. The first is to gain additional length to reach distal or multiple distal coronary artery branches. A second, and, we feel, an important, reason is to avoid crossing the midline of the patient, which may be necessary if the right IMA is planned as a graft to the left coronary system. If the patent in situ graft lies anterior to the heart and just beneath the sternum, reentry during a redo operation without injury to the graft may

From Grooters RK and Nishida H: (editors): *Alternative Bypass Conduits and Methods for Surgical Coronary Revascularization.* © Futura Publishing Co., Inc., Armonk, NY, 1994.

be impossible. If the graft is posterior through the transverse sinus, traction on the heart during dissection in order to gain exposure of the posterior and inferior surfaces of the heart may disrupt the intima of the in situ graft and cause its occlusion and a perioperative infarction. Third, if the origin of the subclavian vessels is demonstrated to have any degree of atherosclerosis proximal to the IMA, this conduit should be used only as a free graft. This would prevent the reported[4] late complications of recurrent postoperative angina due to a subclavian artery stenosis.

Techniques of the Proximal Anastomosis

The proximal anastomosis is obviously extremely important to provide adequate flow into the graft, but surgeons have reported the creation of several alternatives to assure that closure of the graft is not caused by the proximal anastomosis. The most commonly used technique[3] is to construct the proximal anastomosis to the ascending aorta (Fig. 1a) with a continuous 6-0 polypropylene suture. If the IMA is greater than 3 mm, this technique is appropriate. A smaller IMA or a thickened ascending aorta prevents this technique from being successful. The technique of using an SV patch with a suitable side branch and suturing the free IMA graft to a small stump using interrupted 7-0 sutures has been successful.[5] The hood of an SV graft, as Barner[6] described, is also very convenient to use (Fig. 1b).

Another simple, readily available technique is to use autologous pericardium[7] as a patch on the ascending aorta (Fig. 1c). Tector and colleagues[8] have reported anastomosing the free IMA graft to the proximal in situ IMA as a Y graft to gain length (Chapter 8). By creating this composite graft, more coronary vessels can be bypassed, and manipulation of the calcified ascending aorta can be avoided. An end-to-end extension graft that provides additional arterial conduit length to revascularize multiple vessels on the posterior aspect of the heart is another method reported by Gold and associates[9] (Fig. 2). With this technique, the IMA grafts need to be at least 2 mm in diameter at the distal end of the in situ graft to assure a free flow of greater than 150 cc/min.

Finally, we have also reported the free IMA graft to be used as a coronary-coronary bypass graft (Fig. 2 in Chapter 20) in a patient with no venous conduit.[10] In this situation, the proximal coronary ar-

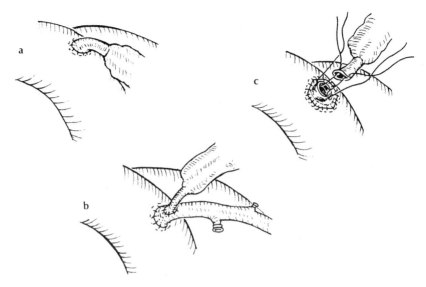

Fig. 1. Three methods of proximal anastomotic construction for the free graft. In this series by Loop and associates,[3] all proximal anastomoses were made directly into the aorta (a). Alternative techniques are useful when there is aortic atherosclerosis, or the IMA is small. These include a vein patch at the site of a side branch and grafting the IMA into the hood of a vein graft (from Loop FD, et al.[3]).

tery feeding the free graft needs to be free of disease and of significant size, 2 mm or greater, to provide sufficient inflow to the graft.

Clinical Results

By far, the largest experience with the free IMA graft technique has been reported by the Cleveland Clinic.[3] From 1971 to 1985, 156 patients received 166 free IMA grafts in the aortocoronary position. Eighty-one percent of the patients were men. The mean age was 54 years, with a range of 33 to 73 years. Bilateral SV stripping had been performed in 44 patients (28%), and reoperations were excluded. Both the left and right IMAs were used as free grafts, and patency rates remained stable after 18 months (Table 1).

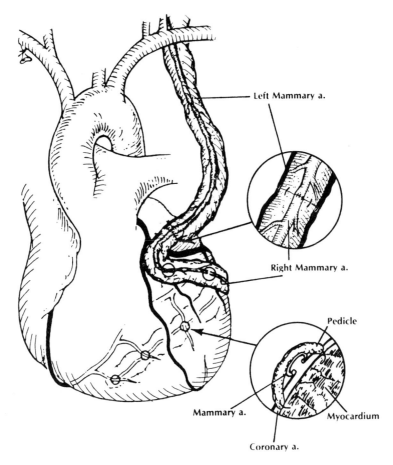

Fig. 2. The completed revascularization, demonstrating the five distal mammary artery-coronary artery anastomoses and the end-to-end distal left mammary artery-proximal right mammary artery anastomosis (from Gold JP, et al.[9]).

Only one hospital death occurred as a result of a myocardial infarction. Respiratory dysfunction defined as intubation for more than 24 hours or the occurrence of pneumothorax, pneumonia, reintubation, or prolonged pulmonary physiotherapy was the most frequent complication occurring in 16 patients (10%). Reoperation for persistent bleeding occurred in 13 patients (8%) and was the second most-frequent complication. Four patients (3%) had strokes. Only three

Table 1
Patency Rates of 75 Free IMA Grafts

	≤ 18 mo.	>18 mo.	> 60 mo.
Studied	40	35	26
Patent	31 (77%)	32 (91%)	24 (92%)

From Loop FD, et al.[3]

patients (2%) developed a new Q-wave myocardial infarction, and two of the patients (1%) experienced wound infections.

Postoperative angiography was conducted on 71 patients; in 33 patients it was done for routine follow-up, and in the remainder for recurrence of symptoms. Of the 75 free IMA grafts restudied at a mean interval of 94 months, 63 (84%) were patent. Long-term patency remained excellent. Grafts to any of the coronary arteries maintained excellent patency rates and, of those free grafts that were patent, none showed evidence of graft atherosclerosis. The most gratifying finding was that of the 26 free IMA grafts studied 5 or more years postoperatively 24 (92%) were patent (Table 1).

Of the 155 patients who survived the operation, the mean follow-up was 98 months. There were 31 late deaths. One hundred sixteen patients were available for follow-up analysis. Of these, 72 patients (62%) remained in NYHA Class I, 33 (28%) in Class II, 6 (5%) in Class III, and 5 (4%) in Class IV. The actuarial five- and ten-year survival rates were 90.2% and 73.0% respectively. Only eight patients (7.0%) underwent another cardiac operation during the follow-up period, seven for coronary bypass and one for aortic valve replacement.

Summary

The free IMA graft appears to be an excellent addition to the surgeon's armamentarium. The graft maintains its resistance to the development of atherosclerosis. This may be, in part, due to the fact that the nourishment of the media comes entirely from the lumen, thus suggesting that harvesting and disconnecting the mammary as a free graft would not result in ischemic injury.[11] Unique vasoactive and anatomical properties previously summarized in Chapter 1 are probably responsible for additional resistance to atherosclerotic development. Most important, the late results of the free IMA graft reported by Loop,[3] demonstrating a 92% patency rate at 5 years or more, provides excellent support for considering either mammary artery as a free graft to any coronary artery, provided the proximal anastomosis is properly constructed to assure good graft inflow.

References

1. Loop FD, Effler DB, Spampinato N, Groves LK, et al. Myocardial revascularization by internal mammary artery graft: a technique without optical assistance. J Thorac Cardiovasc Surg 1972; 63:674.
2. Loop FD, Spampinato H, Cheanvechai C, Effler DB. The free internal mammary artery bypass graft. Ann Thorac Surg 1973; 15:50–55.
3. Loop FD, Lytle BW, Cosgrove DM, Golding LA, et al. Free (aorta-coronary) internal mammary artery graft. J Thorac Cardiovasc Surg 1986; 92:827–831.
4. Olsen CO, Dunton RF, Maggs PR, Lakey SJ. Review of coronary-subclavian steal following internal mammary artery-coronary artery bypass surgery. Ann Thorac Surg 1988; 46:675–678.
5. Schimert G, Vidne BA, Lee AB Jr. Free internal mammary artery graft: an improved surgical technique. Ann Thorac Surg 1975; 19:474–477.
6. Barner, HB. The internal mammary artery as a free graft. J Thorac Cardiovasc Surg 1973: 66:219–221.
7. Kanter KR, Barner HB. Improved technique for the proximal anastomosis with free internal mammary artery grafts. Ann Thorac Surg 1987; 44:556–557.
8. Tector AJ, Schmahl TM, Canino VR. Expanding the use of the internal mammary artery to improve patency in coronary artery bypass grafting. J Thorac Cardiovasc Surg 1986; 91:9–16.
9. Gold JP, Shemen RJ, DiSesa VJ, Cohn L, et al. Multiple-vessel coronary revascularization with combined in situ and free sequential internal mammary arteries. J Thorac Cardiovasc Surg 1985; 90:301–302.
10. Nishida H, Soltanzadeh H, Grooters RK, Thieman KC. Coronary-coronary bypass using internal mammary artery. Ann Thorac Surg 1988; 46:577–578.
11. Landymore RW, Chapman DM. Anatomical studies to support the extended use of the internal mammary artery for myocardial revascularization. Ann Thorac Surg 1987; 44:4–7.

15

The Composite Graft

Ronald K. Grooters and Hiroshi Nishida

With increasing frequency, cardiac surgeons will be faced with inadequate venous or arterial conduits and severely atherosclerotic ascending aortas. Previous bypass surgery will usually be responsible for the lack of routine conduit availability, but previous vein stripping and, occasionally, the patient's poor venous or arterial conduit development will continue to challenge the surgeon's ingenuity. As coronary revascularization is conducted on the elderly patient with increasing frequency, the diseased ascending aorta with [1] friable intraluminal debris or [2] liquid, pastelike intramural atheromatous material will more often be encountered. These conditions are treacherous because emboli complications such as stroke[2] and "trash heart"[3] from clamping or manipulation of the diseased structure are significantly increased. Placement of the proximal anastomoses may also be difficult or impossible or result in technical failure. Techniques such as bilateral internal mammary artery (IMA) grafting (Chapter 12), a "no-touch" technique,[4] including the right gastroepiploic artery (RGEA), sequential grafting, innominate artery-coronary artery venous grafting (Chapter 18), subclavian artery-coronary artery venous grafting (Chapter 19), and coronary-coronary artery grafting (Chapter 20), may aid surgeons with these challenges, but occasionally composite techniques also merit consideration to safely complete myocardial revascularization.

Certain composite variations may become increasingly attractive alternatives, particularly if surgeons discover that this part of their armamentarium can provide reliable, long-term benefits. Although no large studies have been reported, good outcomes may be possible

From Grooters RK and Nishida H: (editors): *Alternative Bypass Conduits and Methods for Surgical Coronary Revascularization.* © Futura Publishing Co., Inc., Armonk, NY, 1994.

if arterial components such as the RGEA, the inferior epigastric artery (IEA), or in the future, perhaps the radial artery (RA) are used with the IMA to form an atherosclerotic resistance-arterial composite. This is not to say that vein segments have no place—they do—but surgeons will need to consider the patient's condition as well as their own preference in the selection of conduit used. No matter what conduit material is available or used, proper construction of the graft (without stenoses, kinks, twists, or tension) and adequate coronary "run-off" to viable myocardium will be the main determinants of composite conduit success.

Classification and Description of Methods

Y-Graft Composite

(I) Vein To Artery

Attachment of the saphenous vein (SV) to an IMA in situ has been reported by Peigh and colleagues[5] and Mills and Everson[6] as an appropriate method (Fig. 1) to avoid clamp manipulation of the severely atherosclerotic ascending aorta and thus prevent perioperative stroke. It is necessary to use the femoral artery for arterial perfusion or at least find a "clean" spot remote from the diseased aorta, which may include the transverse arch (Fig. 1 in Chapter 18).[7] Myocardial protection is then provided by profound systemic hypothermia (20°C to 22°C) and by ventricular fibrillation without the crossclamp and cardioplegia. Ventricular venting may be necessary if the heart or the pulmonary artery distend, and occasionally brief periods of total circulatory arrest are needed. If inadequate venous conduit is the primary reason for employing this composite technique, usually routine perfusion has already been planned or instituted. The SV-IMA anastomosis is sutured with 7-0 polypropylene while cooling the patient and before the distal anastomoses are done. Mills and Everson[6] remove a tiny wedge of IMA before constructing the SV-IMA anastomosis (Fig. 2) to facilitate accuracy and prevent a stenosis of the IMA. We are not sure that this is necessary. In our experience, stenoses have not developed at this site, and a probe has always easily passed through the IMA at this point. We do feel that it is necessary to bring the IMA into the surgical field from beneath the sternum and rotate it 180° as illustrated (Fig. 2), which will make it easier to perform this

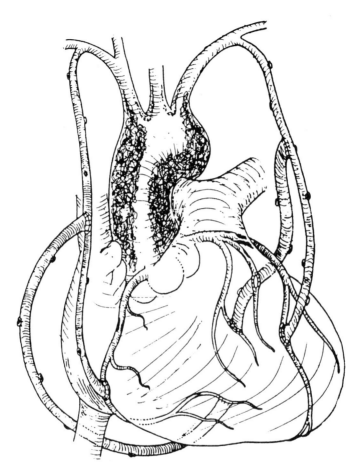

Fig. 1. Bilateral internal mammary artery (IMA) grafts may be used in conjunction with saphenous vein (SV) grafts when the ascending aorta is severely diseased. The SV grafts are anastomosed proximally to the proximal IMA and to the side. (Reprinted with permission from Mills NL. Physiologic and technical aspects of internal mammary artery-coronary artery bypass grafts. In: Cohn LH, ed. Modern Techniques in Surgery: Cardiac/Thoracic Surgery. Mt. Kisco, NY: Futura Publishing Co., 1982:48.17.)

graft connection. Simultaneous free-flow composite measurements through both the IMA graft and the connected vein graft can then be measured after the composite is completed. If poor flow of one of the limbs is detected, corrective measures can be easily accomplished, which may likely include the take down of the anastomoses to redo it.

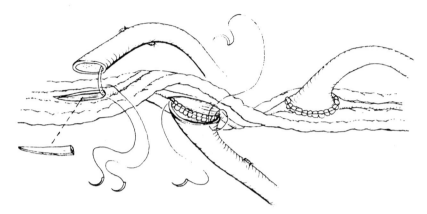

Fig. 2. Anastomoses of the SV grafts to the IMAs are performed with 7-0 polypropylene suture while the patient is rewarmed. SV grafts from the circumflex system are anastomosed to the underside of the left IMA at the level of the first rib. A small wedge of IMA is removed. The length of the arteriotomy is at least twice the diameter of the SV grafts. SV grafts from across the anterior cardiac surface are anastomosed to the anterior side of the IMA (from Mills NL, et al.[6]).

Of the 16 patients reported by Mills and Everson[6] in whom this technique was used to construct 26 SV-IMA end-to-side anastomoses, there were no strokes and 2 unrelated deaths. They have also illustrated bringing a venous limb off the RGEA to assure complete revascularization of the inferior wall of the heart (Fig. 3). The RGEA flow was not reported, but the in situ IMA free flow ranged from 130 to 420 mL/min. This high flow is very important to assure enough perfusion reserve to a larger vascular bed. Postoperative angiography performed on 6 patients revealed no IMA closures and 12 out of 13 SV-IMA anastomoses widely patent up to 3 years postoperatively. Peigh and colleagues[5] used the same composite techniques on nine out of ten patients (six with calcified aortas and four with aortic dissections) without operative mortality and had one transient stroke without sequelae. Nine patients are still doing well at a mean follow-up period of 4 years. One patient died of unknown causes 4 years postoperatively. No angiographic follow-up was reported.

We have used this technique because of inadequate venous conduit on four patients. All had normal treadmill tests 2 to 3 months postoperatively, and 1 patient was studied 6 months postoperatively

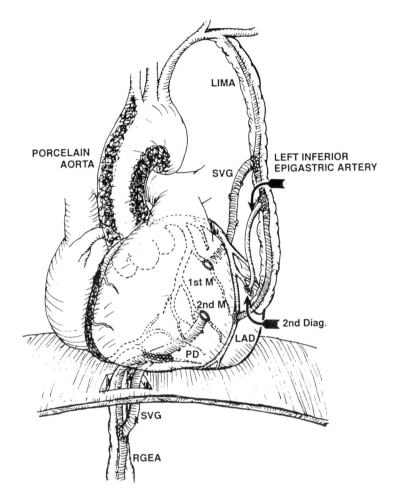

Fig. 3. Operation using a "no-touch" technique for ascending aortic disease. SV grafts are anastomosed to the IMAs and the RGEA after hypothermic cardiac fibrillation is used with low blood flow or circulatory arrest. The right IMA is not used in diabetic patients because of the significantly increased chance of sternal infection with the use of double IMA grafts. Abbreviations: LIMA: left internal mammary artery; SVG: saphenous vein graft; M: marginal; PD: posterior descending (from Mills NL, et al.[6]).

because of symptoms. This last patient's composite graft demonstrated patency of both limbs (Fig. 4), and the cause of the symptoms was of noncardiac etiology.

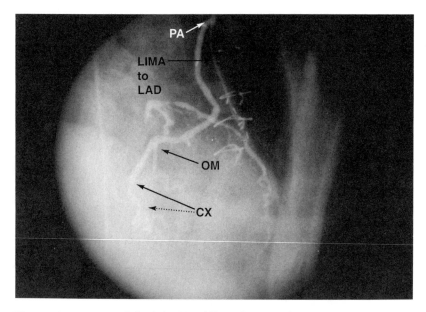

Fig. 4. Angiogram of the left IMA filling the Y graft-vein segment going to the obtuse margin and circumflex. Abbreviations: PA: proximal anastomoses of vein graft; OM: obtuse marginal; CX: circumflex.

(II) Artery To Vein

This type of Y-graft composite (Fig. 5) is not as attractive since the free arterial segment (atherosclerotic resistant) patency may be at risk from acute closure or atherosclerotic development of the venous segment proximal to the arterial-vein/end-to-side anastomosis. Nevertheless, when the SV was thin walled and without phlebosclerosis, we have used this technique in three patients when the in-situ IMA graft was, by nature, too short or needed to be shortened because of disease or injury and would not reach the ascending aorta as a free graft without tension. If the arterial segment has a large diameter (2 mm or greater), we would rather graft important vessels such as the left anterior descending (LAD) or a large obtuse marginal with this limb rather than use another vein segment or include the additional coronary artery in a sequential vein graft. Consideration does need to be given if other possible arterial conduits are available to provide additional length to the short arterial segment as an end-to-end composite or to create an arterial-arterial Y graft. We have not

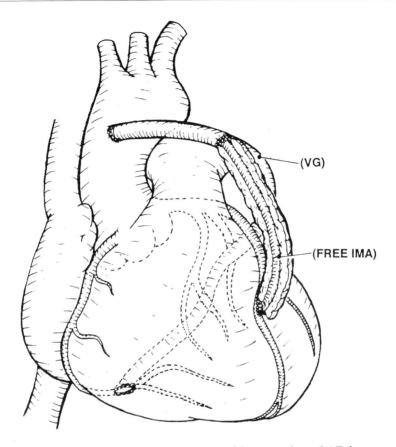

Fig. 5. The very short IMA graft segment able to reach an LAD by means of Y grafting to a normal SV graft, which is then used to bypass the CX and PD arteries.

angiographically studied this composite, but none of the patients have developed postoperative angina or ischemia with treadmill testing.

(III) Vein To Vein

In the period before extensive IMA usage, we occasionally used this composite Y graft when venous conduits of adequate length were not present because of multiple narrowed phlebitic segments throughout the saphenous system or previous harvest. In the last 5 years (1987–1992), we have used this technique in two elderly patients who required emergency surgery. Severe atherosclerosis of both IMAs contraindicated their usage. Segments of SV 20 cm each in length were all that could be found. Remaining venous segments were sclerotic and narrowed. These 2 patients have done well and are alive 3 and 4 years later. One patient had angiography 6 months postoperatively (Fig. 6). The main vein graft (15 cm long) was used to revascularize the LAD and the shorter vein graft was anastomosed to the midportion of the LAD graft with each limb of the Y graft used to revascularize the circumflex (CX) and posterior descending (PD) arteries.

(IV) Artery To Artery

The IMA Y graft composite is frequently being used and is preferred in many cases (Chapters 12 and 14) so that the right IMA conduit can be extended without tension to graft the frequently inaccessible lateral and posterior coronary arteries. Other arterial conduits have been reported as Y graft material. Mills and Everson[6] have brought the left IEA off the in situ left IMA to bypass a diagonal coronary artery (Fig. 3). This was part of a myocardial revascularization procedure to avoid an atherosclerotic aorta. Tanimoto and colleagues[8] have recently used two free segments of RGEA to graft a diagonal and a posterolateral branch of the CX. Saphenous veins (SVs) were not usable, and the left IMA was hard and not feasible for grafting. Postoperative arteriography showed the patency of all grafts (Fig. 7). This technique demonstrated the versatility provided by the RGEA when an alternative is needed if conventional conduits are unsuitable.

End-To-End Composites

(I) Vein To Artery

Only two case reports describe the use of this type of composite. Brodman and Robinson[9] described a patient with previous bypass surgery and a previous stripping of the right greater SV. Only a limited amount of left SV was available. During the procedure, because of a very friable aorta denuded of adventitia during the previous bypass operation, an aortic tear developed at the cannulation site, and

(A)

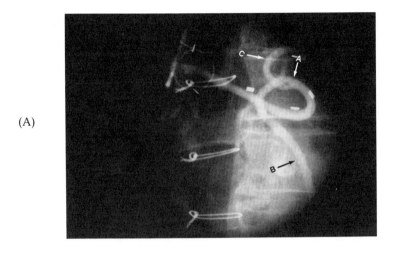

(B)

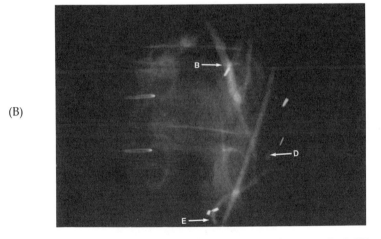

Fig. 6. Illustration of Y grafting using a segment of vein to the LAD and the short bifurcated vein segment to the vessels on the lateral and inferior surfaces of the heart. The Y graft does not reach the ascending aorta for the proximal anastomosis. A—proximal anastomosis of the Y-vein graft onto the LAD vein graft; B—LAD vein graft; C—proximal limb of the Y graft; D— distal anastomosis of one limb of the Y graft to an OM (barely visible); E—other distal limb to a CX (although barely visible, it is nicely patent).

profuse bleeding required femoral cannulation. Proximal anastomoses were performed on the ascending aorta, but upon removal of the clamp, a transverse tear of the aorta developed at the site of vein

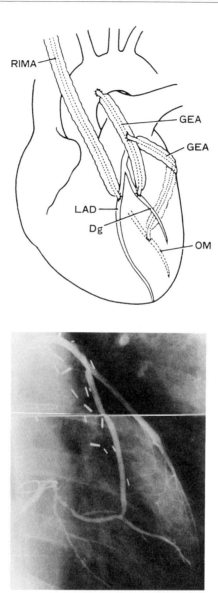

Fig. 7. Coronary arteriogram in the right anterior oblique projection. The free gastroepiploic artery was grafted to the diagonal and OM branches to form a Y graft. The illustration (top) shows the right internal mammary artery (RIMA) grafted to the LAD with the GEA and the graft to the diagonal and OM. (from Tanimoto Y, et al.[8]).

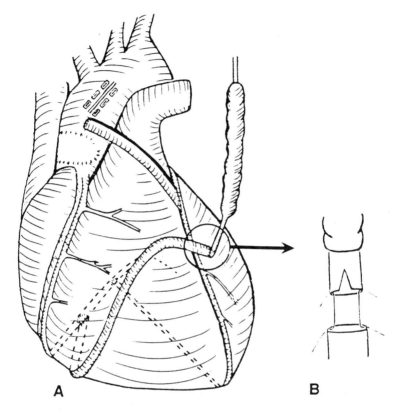

Fig. 8. (A) Left IMA-SV bypass to the distal RCA. SV bypass from the aorta to the LAD. Patch and repair of the arterial cannulation site on the ascending aorta. (B) Technique used to enlarge the circumference of the IMA for the end-to-end anastomosis to the SV graft (from Brodman R, et al.[9]).

graft origin of the new graft to the RCA. Repair necessitated removal of this graft from the aorta and pericardial patch repair of the aortic defect. It was then elected to harvest the left IMA and anastomose the distal end of the IMA to the proximal end of the SV graft (Fig. 8A). Spatulation of the IMA as depicted (Fig. 8B) was necessary to facilitate the anastomosis. Several options were entertained to deal with the SV graft, but this type of composite was felt to be the safest. Coronary angiography showed the patency of the IMA-SV composite anastomoses three weeks postoperatively.

Murphy and Hatcher[10] used this technique to avoid instrumentation of a severely calcified aorta from the annulus extending 2 cm onto the innominate artery. The left IMA was not of sufficient length to reach the large 2.0 mm CX directly. A segment of reversed SV was anastomosed to the CX and, upon rewarming the patient, the end-to-end anastomosis was constructed between the spatulated ends of the IMA and the SV. The patient made an uneventful recovery, and angiography revealed a patent graft. The patient was asymptomatic 3 months after discharge.

(II) Artery To Vein

No such composite has been reported. It is difficult to conceive of any circumstance that would necessitate this combination. Obviously, other alternatives provide the solutions that surgeons need.

(III) Vein To Vein

This alternative is also not found in the literature, but we have used it when the inadequate length of vein segments is the problem. If the IMA graft flows are poor (< 50 mL/min), we have preferred to splice available short, but normal, SV segments to one another to achieve adequate length rather than use an SV-IMA Y graft composite. The ends of the SV segments are spatulated, and 7-0 polypropylene continuous suture is used. After the splicing is finished, a large probe (2.5 mm or greater) is passed through the graft to detect a possible anatomical stenosis. The distal coronary anastomoses are then routinely performed, and during rewarming the proximal anastomosis is then constructed to the ascending aorta with 5-0 polypropylene. Other alternatives are given consideration before this simple technique is reluctantly used.

(IV) Artery To Artery

The direct end-to-end arterial composite has been reported with success using a free IMA[11] and an IEA[12] as the extension of an in situ IMA to provide a complete coronary revascularization. This alternative is indicated if SV conduit is not available or the ascending aorta is severely diseased. Gold et al.[11] used the free IMA composite to provide a sequence of five anastomoses in a patient with severe multivessel disease without adequate venous conduit (Fig. 2 in Chapter

14). The IMA grafts used were of adequate diameter (2.0–2.5 mm) throughout the entire length. This technique was used to correct the "coronary steal" phenomenon following the first attempt to provide flow to the free graft from the proximal LAD because the IMA free graft was too short for an aorta-IMA anastomosis. The patient did well, and angiography 1 week postoperatively demonstrated all of the anastomoses to be patent. Buche and colleagues[12] applied the IMA-IEA composite to five patients without suitable veins. Four patients underwent postoperative angiography showing all grafts patent with good flow. The fifth patient refused angiography but had a negative stress test at 6 weeks.

The principles of this technique are similar to any end-to-end anastomoses. The suturing is best completed with 7-0 or 8-0 polypropylene before the distal coronary anastomoses are constructed. It was suggested that at least a 1.5 mm caliber at the distal end of the feeding artery is necessary to provide adequate inflow. Each end is longitudinally split a length of 5 mm before anastomosed together. The free flow can then be measured. The accompanying pedicle of tissue (veins and muscle) of the distal component should be sutured to the distal end of the feeding vessel pedicle. This will reinforce the fragile anastomosis and keep it from twisting (Fig. 2 in Chapter 14). If arterial conduits other than the IMA (i.e., the RGEA or IEA) are used as the extension, it is prudent, if possible, to limit their use to bypass a myocardial segment of less value or vessels that cannot be safely and technically reached by an IMA graft. The Y graft artery-to-artery composite should always be considered as an alternative to this end-to-end composite. With the Y graft, the anastomoses of the free-graft extension are located proximally on the feeding vessel at a point of larger diameter and, thus, should provide higher blood flows than an end-to-end composite.

Comment

It is understandable that surgeons may feel uncomfortable with composite grafting because of the added anastomosis in the mainstream of a reconstructed conduit, which may jeopardize all of the downstream bypasses. The increased risk of acute thrombosis may be present, but it has not been specifically reported. Yet, if confronted with an increased risk of stroke from a severely diseased ascending aorta or a lack of satisfactory conduit, the versatility of these techniques certainly justify their use. In general, composite grafts are still considered alternatives, but as the free IMA graft gains favor, the Y-IMA-IMA composite may become a routine option for providing a complete arterial myocardial revascularization. In conclusion, although the composite can be a successful alternative, it should not be considered as a substitute for the various techniques discussed in this book but only as another good alternative for selective situations.

References

1. Coselli JS, Crawford ES. Aortic valve replacement in the patient with extensive calcification of the ascending aorta (the porcelain aorta). J Thorac Cardiovasc Surg 1986; 91:184–187.
2. Gardner TJ, Horneffer PJ, Manolio TA, Pearson TA, et al. Stroke following coronary artery bypass grafting: a ten-year study. Ann Thorac Surg 1985; 40:574–581.
3. Keon WJ, Heggtveit HA, Leduc J. Perioperative myocardial infarction caused by atheroembolism. J Thorac Cardiovasc Surg 1982; 84:849–855.
4. Suma H. Coronary artery bypass grafting in patients with calcified ascending aorta: aortic no-touch technique. Ann Thorac Surg 1989; 48: 728–730.
5. Peigh PS, DeSesa VJ, Collins JJ Jr, Cohn LH. Coronary bypass grafting with totally calcified or acutely dissected ascending aorta. Ann Thorac Surg 1991; 51:102–104.
6. Mills NL, Everson CT. Atherosclerosis of the ascending aorta and coronary artery bypass: pathology, clinical correlates, and operative management. J Thorac Cardiovasc Surg 1991; 102:546–553.
7. Holland DL, Hieb RE. Revascularization without embolization: coronary bypass in the presence of a calcified aorta. Ann Thorac Surg 1985; 40:308–310.
8. Tanimoto Y, Matsuda Y, Masuda T, Sakota K, et al. Multiple free (aorta-coronary) gastroepiploic artery grafting. Ann Thorac Surg 1990; 49: 479–480.
9. Brodman R, Robinson G. Internal mammary artery-saphenous vein composite conduit: an alternative for the proximal coronary anastomosis. Ann Thorac Surg 1981; 31:370–372.
10. Murphy DA, Hatcher CR Jr. Coronary revascularization in the presence of ascending aortic calcification: use of an internal mammary artery-saphenous vein composite graft. J Thorac Cardiovasc Surg 1984; 86: 789–791.
11. Gold JP, Shemin RJ, DiSesa VJ, Cohn LH, et al. Multiple-vessel coronary revascularization with combined in-situ and free sequential internal mammary arteries. J Thorac Cardiovasc Surg 1985; 90:301–302.
12. Buche M, Schroeder E, Devaux P, Louazie YAG, et al. Right internal mammary artery extended with an inferior epigastric artery for circumflex and right coronary bypass. Ann Thorac Surg 1992; 54:381–383.

16

Coronary Bypass Using the Inverted Internal Mammary Artery

Ronald K. Grooters and Hiroshi Nishida

The internal mammary artery (IMA) collateralizes distally with the iliac artery through the epigastric artery and also through the musculophrenic and low intercostal arteries from the descending aorta. The retrograde flow from these arteries into the IMA may occasionally be enough to supply a segment of myocardium. This alternative method has been successfully done in one patient.[1] Also, canine studies[2,3] have demonstrated the flow of this technique to be adequate. It has been suggested[1] that in highly selective circumstances this inverted IMA may be considered, but many alternatives reported and suggested in this book are superior.

The Clinical Experience

In 1982, Goiti and Smith[1] reported the first and maybe the only usage of the inverted IMA grafting technique in man. This 56-year-old diabetic patient did not have enough suitable leg vein and had no arm veins. The coronary angiogram demonstrated severe triple-vessel occlusions. When surgery was performed, only 12 cm of leg vein could be found. Both IMAs were mobilized. The left IMA was used antegrade to the left anterior descending (LAD), the vein segment went to the obtuse marginal (OM) artery, and the right IMA was detached proximally from the subclavian artery and used retro-

From Grooters RK and Nishida H: (editors): *Alternative Bypass Conduits and Methods for Surgical Coronary Revascularization.* © Futura Publishing Co., Inc., Armonk, NY, 1994.

grade to bypass the posterior descending (PD) coronary artery. No flow measurements were reported. Eighteen days after the operation, the patient had myocardial imaging using thallium-201. This demonstrated a fixed lateral defect compatible with the previous myocardial infarction but no inferior wall defect. No angina developed. Coronary angiography showed the left IMA to be patent, but the right IMA graft could not be visualized by injecting the inferior epigastric artery. The patient was pain free 8 months after operation.

Experimental Findings

The applicability of this technique in bypassing the distal right coronary artery (RCA)[2] and the circumflex coronary artery (CX)[3] has been experimentally examined in the canine model.

Florian and colleagues[2] used six mongrel dogs to evaluate the right IMA inverted graft as a long-term conduit to the distal RCA. Electrocardiographic (EKG) S-T segment changes and the surface pH of the myocardium were observed and measured to determine myocardial ischemic changes at the time of surgery. The average free retrograde flow from the right IMA graft was also measured and ranged from 10–52 mL/min, with a mean of 24, while the antegrade flow from the left IMA measured at the same time ranged from 100 to 350 mL/min, with a mean of 190. After the inverted graft was constructed, the native RCA was ligated. Once the myocardium was graft dependent, 10 minutes of graft occlusion dropped the surface pH from 7.9–8.1 down to 6.6–7.3, and the S-T segments became elevated an average of 19 mm. After the graft was reopened, the pH normalized, and the EKG S-T segments reverted back to a baseline of 2 mm. The four long-term survivors (6 weeks) were studied angiographically. Two grafts were patent, and two were occluded. Autopsy studies of the two dogs with occluded grafts demonstrated patent anastomoses, but thrombosis had occurred at the angle of graft takeoff from the chest wall.

Folts and colleagues[3] studied retrograde flow of the left IMA that was anastomosed to the CX (a dominant vessel) in 16 dogs. Eight dogs had no prior ligation of the left IMA at the subclavian artery origin (Group I), and in eight dogs the left IMA was ligated (Group II). The anastomoses were cleverly done with a stent in the CX during the suturing of the anastomosis and without cardiopulmonary bypass. The average free flow in Group I was 39 ± 24 mL/min and in Group II was 71 ± 22 mL/min. Average electromagnetic flow-meter measurements were 24 ± 11 mL/min in Group I and 39 ± 12 mL/min in Group II after completion of the anastomosis. No "steal" phenomena were detected in either group. All grafts were patent, and retrograde flow seemed adequate to maintain perfusion of the myocardium as evidenced by EKG and hemodynamic stability.

Human Flow Study

Cohen and associates[4] studied the retrograde flow of the IMA in 32 patients undergoing coronary artery bypass. After dividing the IMA 5 mm proximal to the distal bifurcation, both the antegrade flow from the IMA graft and the retrograde flow of the distal stump were allowed to bleed freely and measured for 30 seconds. The mean antegrade flow from the IMA graft was 73 ± 34 mL/min, and the stump retrograde flow was 25 ± 17 mL/min ($P < 0.05$). These researchers concluded that a retrograde IMA graft should not be recommended as a primary form of myocardial revascularization. In selective circumstances, if adequate retrograde flow is present, this technique may be considered.

Conclusion

The retrograde IMA bypass method appears to provide adequate myocardial blood flow to at least one coronary artery. This grafting technique cannot be angiographically studied, and the graft may also thrombose at its angled takeoff from the chest wall. Today, other alternative techniques and conduits provide better flow rates and are more practical. It is difficult to imagine a condition existing in which this grafting technique is the alternative of choice.

References

1. Goiti JJ, Smith GH. Coronary artery surgery using inverted internal mammary artery. Br Heart J 1982; 48:81–82.
2. Florian A, Lamberti JJ, Cohn LH, Collins JJ. Revascularization of the right coronary artery by retrograde perfusion of the mammary artery: an experimental study. J Thorac Cardiovasc Surg 1975; 70:19–23.
3. Folts JD, Gallagher KP, Kroncke GM, Rowe GG. Myocardial revascularization of the canine circumflex coronary artery using retrograde internal mammary artery flow without cardiopulmonary bypass. Ann Thorac Surg 1981; 31:21–27.
4. Cohen AJ, Ameika JA, Briggs RA, Grishkin BA, et al. Retrograde flow in the internal mammary artery. Ann Thorac Surg 1988; 45:48–49.

Part V
Alternative
Bypass Methods
Using the
Saphenous Vein

Chapter 17

Sequential Vein Grafting

Ronald K. Grooters and Hiroshi Nishida

Multiple sequential grafting of coronary arteries using a single segment of reversed saphenous vein (SV) was initially reported by Flemma and colleagues[1] in 1971. The enthusiasm for this technique soon became apparent when Bartley and his group[2] revascularized the entire myocardium using a long segment of SV (Fig. 1). This became known as the "snake graft,"[3] or circular graft,[4] and other authors labeled this technique a "jump graft."[5,6] Cheanvechai and coworkers at the Cleveland Clinic[7] did not agree with the concept of grafting all three major coronary arteries with one vein graft, but used the technique in a limited fashion as a "bridge graft" to bypass a minor branch and a major branch (i.e., aorta to diagonal and left anterior descending (LAD) coronary artery. The advantages of sequential grafting became evident over time. In 1981, Brower and colleagues[8] reported shorter operating and ischemic arrest times. Other surgeons[9,10] felt that a more complete revascularization could be made by including otherwise frequently neglected smaller coronary arteries. Also, less venous conduit was used, which saved conduit for other vascular procedures or redo coronary operations. Meurala and associates[11] reported that both early and late patency rates were better with sequential grafts (95%) than with a single graft (80%), although other authors found no differences.[3,8] The flow velocity of the proximal segment of the SV graft was found to be higher than the single vein grafts,[12-14] which was felt to enhance the patency of the vein graft, yet the total blood flow was less with the sequential technique than with multiple single venous bypass grafts. This was found not to adversely influence the clinical outcomes of operative

From Grooters RK and Nishida H: (editors): *Alternative Bypass Conduits and Methods for Surgical Coronary Revascularization.* © Futura Publishing Co., Inc., Armonk, NY, 1994.

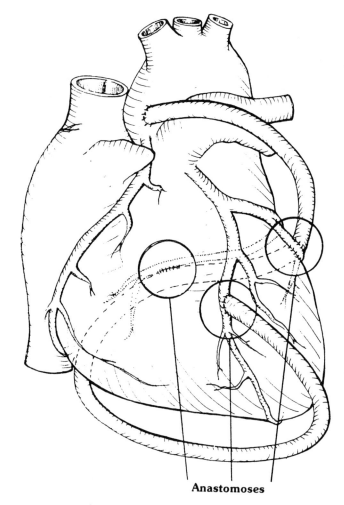

Anastomoses

Fig. 1. Aortocoronary bypass with multiple anastomoses with a single vein first reported by Bartley.[2] (from Bartley TD, et al.[2]).

mortality or symptom relief. Additionally, the technical aspect of constructing only one proximal anastomosis is very helpful when a very small or diseased ascending aorta is encountered.

The argument against the use of total revascularization with a vein graft based on one proximal anastomosis is a valid one today. Now the questions of when and to what extent this technique should be used are even more important since the internal mammary artery (IMA) and other arterial conduits give both superior short- and long-term results. The technical aspects of the sequential technique have mostly been clarified and described,[4,7,9,15,16] but whether or not sequential grafting for a particular case is used as an alternative or an adjunct in myocardial revascularization may be more a matter of judgment than science or dogma.

Methodology and Technique

In general, the use of grafts and grafting methods is planned on the basis of the angiographic and ventriculogram findings prior to the operation. Whether sequential grafts are an option will first depend on the number of vessels identified as requiring bypass grafting. Significant tandem blockages within the same artery are ideal for bridge grafts (Fig. 2). The size of the coronary arteries and the amount of myocardium in jeopardy supplied by a particular vessel or group of vessels will also influence our choices of conduit and technique. If the ventriculogram is normal, we will use sequential grafting to the smaller, least important vessels. With an abnormal ventricle, we tend to use sequential vein grafting to vessels supplying hypokinetic or

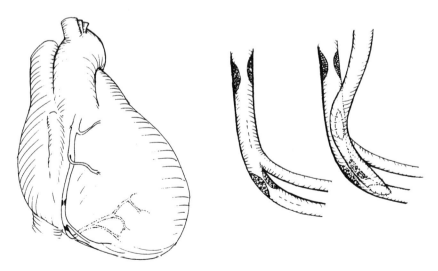

Fig. 2. Right coronary artery (RCA). Diagram of a bridge graft constructed to the atrioventricular branch and main RCA (from Cheanvechai C, et al.[7]).

akinetic myocardial segments and to use IMA grafting for large coronary arteries supplying normal contracting myocardium. For example, in a patient with triple-vessel disease but a hypokinetic anterior wall, a large circumflex (CX) coronary artery and a smaller, moderately sized right coronary artery (RCA), we most likely would bypass the CX with an IMA and use a sequential vein graft technique to the LAD and posterior descending (PD) artery.

We must also be ready to use other methods if coronary atherosclerosis distal to major obstructions and not anticipated from coronary angiography is encountered. Placing a graft (sequential or single) proximal to nonobstructive, early distal disease may not benefit the patient over the long term. We then will more often use separate single vein grafts with splitting of plaque, tandem grafting, or endarterectomy, whichever is applicable. Our whole idea is to use sequential vein grafting to gain from its benefits but not to force the use of this technique when other methods are needed to enhance the long-term benefits of myocardial revascularization.

Distal Anastomosis

Soon after the institution of cardiopulmonary bypass, the entire surface of the heart is inspected to evaluate the coronary artery branches for sites of graft placement. If unexpected distal atherosclerosis is seen and more venous conduit is needed, it can be harvested at this time and preserved in blood as described in Chapter 2. The patient is then cooled (32°C to 34°C), and cardioplegia is given. All venous anastomoses are sutured with continuous 7-0 polypropylene. The sequential technique is usually started with the most proximal side-to-side anastomosis done first. We prefer the "diamond" crossover technique (Fig. 3A) if three or more anastomoses are planned. With this technique, a larger anastomosis can be achieved, which was confirmed by casting models in a study by Shioi and coworkers.[17] A regular side-to-side anastomosis (Fig. 3c) is also commonly used, but a 1–3 mm longitudinal slit is added, particularly if the coronary arteriotomy is a little larger than the transverse venous opening (Fig. 4). Care must always be taken not to open the artery more than a third of the diameter of the vein graft. This will prevent narrowing of the graft at the anastomosis (Fig. 5). If only two anastomoses are planned for the vein graft and plenty of distance between the two

(*text continues on p. 173*)

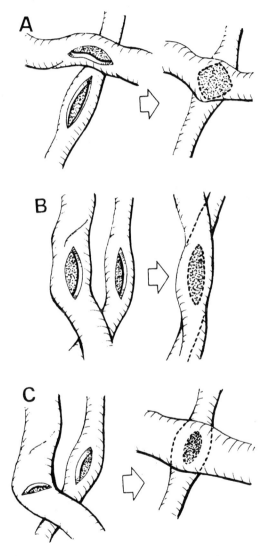

Figure 3. Anastomotic procedures: A—crossed side-to-side anastomosis with longitudinal incision "diamond" anastomosis. B—parallel side-to-side anastomosis with longitudinal incisions. C—crossed side-to-side anastomosis with one longitudinal and one transverse incision (from Shioi K, et al.[17]).

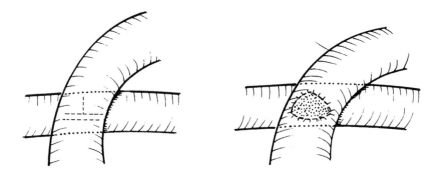

**DIAMOND-SHAPED
SIDE-TO-SIDE ANASTOMOSIS**

Fig. 4. Enlargement of the transverse vein graft incision by using a 1–3 mm perpendicular incision (left) and ending with a modified diamond anastomosis (right).

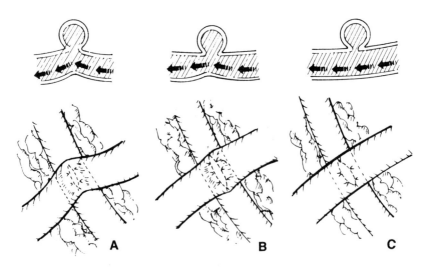

Fig. 5. (A) correct transverse anastomosis. (B) transverse anastomosis made too long. (C) transverse anastomosis made deep in epicardial fat (from Bigelow JC, et al.[21]).

sites permits a smooth curvature to the graft, or if a plaque at the first graft site needs to be split or double jumped, the side-to-side longitudinal technique (Fig. 3b) is preferred.

Sometimes, branches of the vein graft can be used as Y grafts if they are large enough (2.5 mm or more) and can be nicely incorporated with a sequential grafting (Fig. 6). Care must be taken to avoid any twisting or kinking, which we feel is more likely if one of the limbs is not the correct length or is abnormally rotated. A strong injection down the graft after the first limb anastomosis is complete will assist the surgeon in detecting those tendencies or conditions. Veins differ in their tendencies to kink; some have very little curvature, and some veins maintain a very tight curve without developing any occlusive crease.

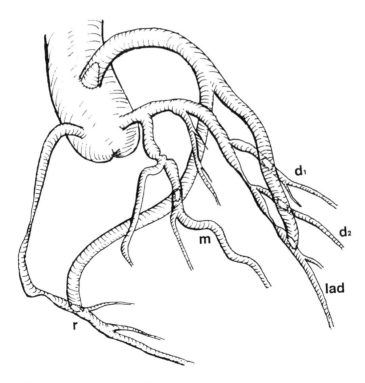

Fig. 6. Aortocoronary quintuple bypass using a bifurcating vein. Abbreviations: d_1—first diagonal; d_2—second diagonal; LAD—left anterior descending; m—obtuse marginal; r—right coronary artery or posterior descending artery (from Yeh TJ, et al.[16]).

Measuring Distances

The distance between two anastomoses must be measured carefully, particularly if the planned anastomoses are close together. This is best accomplished with the vein distended after the proximal anastomosis has been constructed. Then a point on the graft for the second graft site is judged. Care must be taken to observe the fill and contour of the heart as well. If the heart is empty, the distance between the two grafting targets may appear shorter than it really is than when the heart is full and beating. It is usually better to add a small amount of length to the estimated distances. The proximal segment is easier to measure after the crossclamp is released, so the heart can be filled to assess correctly the course of this segment over the pulmonary artery, the size of which can sometimes be underestimated.

Route of the Graft

We nearly always route the graft to the left lateral side of the heart. This will usually keep the proximal segment of the graft away from the substernal area and provide a nice curvature to either a diagonal-LAD or a CX-PD sequential bypass (Fig. 7a). A retroaortic route through the transverse sinus (Fig. 7b) is another option. Seldom do we bring a graft off to the right to lie on the right atrium, and we avoid completely the anterior (substernal) path (Fig. 7c). This discipline evolved to avoid the problem of graft laceration upon re-entry for a redo operation or to avoid embolization from an atherosclerotic vein graft, which we frequently encountered during dissection of an anterior graft for right atrial or ventricular exposure and right atrial cannulation.

Aortic Anastomosis

As a general rule, all the distal anastomoses are completed before the proximal aortic anastomosis is sutured. A continuous suture of 5-0 polypropylene is routinely used. Prior to the release of the crossclamp, the aorta (while soft) is palpated to detect any major atherosclerotic plaque. If plaque is present and it is deemed hazardous to remove the crossclamp and reapply a side clamp, the aorta is opened before release of the crossclamp (Chapter 23, Fig. 8). If no

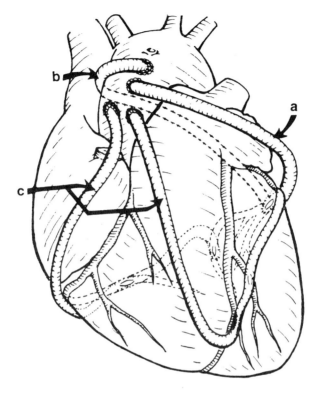

Fig. 7. Vein graft routes. (a) proximal vein segment to the left and lateral. (b) retroaortic route. (c) anterior route; usually avoided to prevent laceration or manipulation upon re-entry during a redo operation.

debris is noted, the proximal anastomosis is constructed during the crossclamp procedure at a place on the ascending aorta that is as normal as possible. If the aorta is normal by palpation, the crossclamp is then removed, and the anastomosis is completed over a side clamp. The aortotomy is nearly always a simple incision, although the punch technique is also acceptable.

Graft Flow Studies

Sequential vein grafts generally have higher blood flows than single vein grafts. This seems logical since the total vascular bed should be larger for the sequential graft. This was obviously demonstrated using the "circular graft"[4] in which flow measurements ranged from 130 to 310 mL/min with 4 to 5 anastomoses patent, whereas most single vein graft flows are 50 ± 20 mL/min, depending on the size of the coronary artery grafted and the resistance of the vascular runoff. McNamara and his colleagues[14] also measured blood flow comparing single, double, and triple sequential grafts. This study demonstrated lesser flows per anastomosis as the number increased (Table 1). Total graft blood flow tended to be higher in sequential grafts, but Harjola and coworkers[18] noted that total blood flow to the heart was higher with multiple single grafts than with sequential grafting. Prioleau and his group[12] also showed that constructing diamond anastomoses with interrupted sutures did not significantly enhance flows for the sequential methods.

In a study of 76 patients, Meurala and colleagues[11] measured blood flow with cineangiographic techniques and, not surprisingly, found the flow between the aorta and the first anastomosis higher than the flow in the control single vein grafts, but the flow decreased between early and late examinations, most rapidly in the distal segment. Concerned about the distal segment, Minale and coworkers[19] compared the blood flow of separate single grafts to the diagonal and the LAD to sequential grafts of the same vessels. They concluded that the LAD was at a higher risk of closure with a sequential graft because of the drop in blood flow of the distal segment. Eschenbruch and associates[5] concluded the opposite based on the finding of higher patency rates (87%) for the distal segments of the sequential graft compared to a single graft patency rate of 82%. They felt that the sequential graft should be planned so that the distal segment of the vein graft should be anastomosed to the vessel with a major flow ca-

Table 1
Blood Flow in Coronary Artery Grafts
Single and Sequential (± SEM)

No. of Distal Anastomoses	No. of Grafts	Total No. Distal Anastomoses	Flow per Graft (cc/min)	Flow per Distal Anastomosis (cc/min)
Single	51	51	85 ± 53 (7.42)	85
Double	76	152	101 ± 50 (5.74)	51
Triple (or more)	13	40	98 ± 40 (11.09)	32

From McNamera JJ, et al.[14]

Table 2
Dimensions of Vein Grafts

	Single Grafts (n = 106)	Sequential Grafts (n = 35)	p Value
Diameter (mm)	4.0 ± 0.05	4.1 ± 0.09	0.535
Length (cm)	17.6 ± 0.42	25.6 ± 0.88	0.001
Arterial pressure (mm Hg)	83 ± 2	83 ± 2	0.984
Hematocrit (%)	22 ± 0.4	22 ± 0.7	0.992
Resistance (RU)*			
Total	190.1 ± 14.7	116.5 ± 15.5	0.001
Graft	15.5 ± 0.7	16.5 ± 1.6	0.531
Coronary	174.6 ± 14.6	100.0 ± 15.6	0.001
Velocity (cc/sec)	7.5 ± 0.6	11.1 ± 1.1	0.003

*RU = dyne · sec · cm^{-5} × 10^{-3}
From O'Neill MJ Jr., et al.[13].

pacity. O'Neill and colleagues[13] measured coronary blood flow at the time of operation in 106 single and 35 sequential grafts. The flow velocity was higher in the proximal segments than in single grafts (Table 2). They also demonstrated improved flow velocity distribution to both coronary arteries if the proximal side-to-side graft was constructed to the smaller coronary artery and the distal segment flowed to a larger coronary system with less vascular resistance (Fig. 8). They concluded that the distal segment be planned for the larger coronary artery. Minale and colleagues,[19] based on this study and their own, believed the opposite. They believed that since the distal segment of the sequential graft had a lower flow rate and patency rate, important coronary arteries such as the LAD should instead be bypassed using single vein grafts.

Reported Clinical Results

Early Procedure Mortality

In the first large reported series of sequential vein grafting, Bartley et al.[2] noted a hospital mortality rate of 6.1% (8 out of 130 patients). Seven of these deaths were in the group of 37 poor-risk pa-

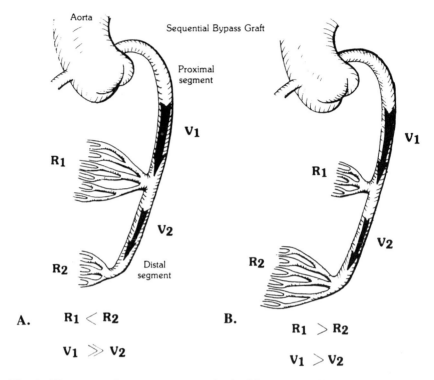

Fig. 8. Diagrammatic representation of a double sequential bypass graft with the proximal anastomosis to the larger coronary artery. (A) The resistance (R_1) of this coronary system is less than the resistance (R_2) of the smaller distal coronary system. The velocity of flow is high in the proximal segment but markedly reduced distally. (B) The order of coronary anastomoses has been reversed in the smaller coronary system (R_2) with less coronary vascular resistance being the distal anastomosis. The velocity of flow in the proximal segment is the same as in (A), but in this instance the velocity of flow to the smaller coronary system is markedly increased when compared to the arrangement illustrated in (A) (from O'Neill, MJ, Jr, et al.[13]).

tients (who had any two of these risk factors: age greater than 60, diastolic blood pressure above 90 mm Hg, diffuse coronary disease, poor ventricular contractility, and left-ventricular end-diastolic pressure above 20 mm Hg). Sewell et al.,[3] using a similar technique of "snake" or "circular" sequential grafting, reported in 1976 a 4.6% early death rate in 227 patients, whereas Cheanvechai et al.,[7] in 1975, and Moreno-Cabral et al.,[15] in 1977, reported low hospital mortality rates of 1.2% and 1.9%, respectively, with the more limited "bridge graft" technique. These mortality rates are no different from those for multiple single-vein grafting. This has now been confirmed by the latest report of Meester and colleagues,[20] in 1991, demonstrating operative mortality rates of 1% for sequential graft usage (234 patients) and 3% for multiple single grafting (284 patients). All of the patients prior to surgery had been symptomatic for angina pectoris and had either triple vessel or left main coronary artery disease.

Perioperative Myocardial Infarction

Using enzyme studies and new Q-wave findings on electrocardiography postoperatively, Cheanvechai et al.,[7] in 1975, reported that 9 (3.6%) out of 250 patients sustained a perioperative myocardial infarction. Moreno-Cabral and colleagues[15] reported a 5% rate in 206 patients. Most other surgeons have not reported their perioperative myocardial infarction rates for sequential grafting.

Distal Anastomotic Patency Rates

In the first report of sequential grafting, Bartley and associates[2] reported 67 out of 87 (77%) distal anastomoses to be patent, but the exact timing of angiographic studies was not stated. This same group of patients was restudied in 1976[21] demonstrating 104 out of 144 (72%) anastomoses patent at 3 years. Numerous studies have assessed patency rates at various postoperative time periods (Table 3), and the latest study by Kieser and coworkers,[10] in 1986, shows an 84% patency rate at 5 years.

Bigelow and colleagues[22] reported a lower patency rate of 60% for single vein grafts at 3 years. In 1982, Meurala and associates[11] reported a comparison of patency rates for single graft versus sequential grafting at a mean of 26 months postoperatively, with results of 80% and 94%, respectively. Sewell et al.,[3] in 1976, reported a patency rate for sequential grafts at 3 months postoperatively of 98%, whereas single- and Y-graft patency rates were 89% and 87%. Yeh and colleagues[16] studied 59 of 425 patients (the 14% representing suboptimal clinical results) and found a Y-graft patency at 93% and both side-to-side and distal end-to-side segments of the sequential graft to be 89% patent. Crosby et al.[23] reported opposite results, with 96% of single vein grafts patent versus 80% of sequential anasto-

Table 3
Patency Rates for Sequential Grafting

Author/ Year	No. of Opera- Tions	Distal Anastomoses Studied	Patent	Percentage Patent	Time Period of Angiogram
Bartley[2]/ 1972*	130	87	67	77%	unknown
Cheanvechi[7]/ 1975	250	220	190	86%	1 mo–2 yrs
Sewell[3]/ 1976	227	504	473	94%	1 mo–3 mos
Bigelow[21]/ 1976*	122	144	104	72%	at 3 yrs
Grondin[9]/ 1977	40 27	96 50	83 47	87% 94%	2 wks 1 yr
Cleveland[4]/ 1980	21	60	58	97%	4–13 mos
Crosby[22]/ 1981	50	80	67	80%	2–3 mos
Meurala[11]/ 1982	76	75	71	94%	26 mos (mean)
Kieser[10]/ 1986	189	212 188 91	205 170 77	96% 91% 84%	early 1 yr 5 yrs

*: the same group reporting

moses patent 2–3 months after surgery. They did state that if defective graft design errors were eliminated, the patency rate for sequential vein grafting was 88%.

Long-Term Survival

In the 1991 report by Meester and coworkers[20], the comparative study of 234 patients in the multiple single-vein graft group and 234 patients in the sequential-vein graft group had a nearly equal probability of survival 5 years postoperatively, 90% and 88%, respectively. At 10 years after surgery, these rates were essentially identical, 71% and 72%, respectively. Although not statistically significant, the multiple single-vein graft group had a higher percentage of cardiac deaths (57%) than did the sequential group (42%). The sequential vein graft patients died of chronic cardiac failure more often, which accounted for 22% of the deaths. Symptomatic relief or improvement from angina pectoris was also similar for both groups: 86% for multiple single grafts and 88% for sequential vein grafts.

Discussion

Cardiac surgeons will always need sequential vein grafting as part of their armamentarium for coronary revascularization. This technique can provide operative advantages such as reduced operating time, shorter ischemic arrest times, and a more complete revascularization for the patient with multiple small-vessel disease. Certain patients with diffuse multiple tandem stenosis are also amenable to sequential grafting (Fig. 2). Added to these advantages is the fact that flow rates and early patency rates are at least equal to, and may be better than, single grafts. These sequential techniques then may be the best alternatives for certain clinical conditions such as catastrophic emergencies from failed percutaneous angioplasty, left ventricular hypertrophy, coronary disease associated with valvular disease, or a postinfarct ventricular septal defect. It may also be the best alternative for the aged (greater than 70 years).

Although the sequential vein grafting technique ("bridge" or "snake" grafting) provides increased flow through at least the proximal segment, which may inhibit acute thrombosis or graft fibrointimal hyperplasia,[11] venous conduits used in this manner apparently are still vulnerable to atherosclerotic changes. The evidence for this may be extrapolated from the lower survival probability at 10 years postoperatively of 71% (when only vein grafts are used),[20,24] but with an IMA bypass to the LAD, the 10-year survival rate improved to 82.6% for those patients with three-vessel disease. We have also noticed atherosclerotic stenosis in every segment of the old (5 years or more) sequential graft when restudied angiographically or observed at reoperation. These lesions are as frequent in the high-flow proximal segment as they are in the low-flow distal segment. No doubt, harvested vein segments are now handled better to prevent ischemic and mechanical damage than they were a few years ago, which may improve long-term patency. Still, the strong fact remains that the IMA and other arterial conduits show better resistance to atherosclerosis. Fujiwara and colleagues[21] have also demonstrated, when comparing peak diastolic velocity in sequential vein grafts (26.3 ± 5.5cm/sec) to IMA grafts (26.6 ± 2.0 cm/sec), that the IMA graft with its smaller diameter will have a higher shear rate. This may provide an additional factor for the superior long-term patency of the IMA graft over sequential vein grafting.

In conclusion, sequential vein grafting is just as effective as multiple single vein grafts and may be the alternative of choice in certain clinical conditions. This technique also conserves SV conduit. When the IMA is available, sequential vein grafting is then more appropriately used as an adjunct for the remaining "less important" graftable coronary arteries.

References

1. Flemma RJ, Johnson WD, Lepley D Jr. Triple aortocoronary vein bypass as treatment for coronary insufficiency. Arch Surg 1971; 103:82–83.
2. Bartley TD, Bigelow JC, Page US. Aortocoronary bypass grafting with multiple sequential anastomosis to a single vein. Arch Surg 1972; 105:915–917.
3. Sewell WH, Sewell KV. Technique for the coronary snake graft operation. Ann Thorac Surg 1976; 22:58–65.
4. Cleveland JC, Lebenson IM, Twokey RJ, Ellis JG, et al. Further evaluation of the circular sequential vein graft technique of coronary artery bypass. Ann Thorac Surg 1980; 30:336–341.
5. Eschenbruch EM, Pabst F, Tolleneare P, Roskamm H, et al. The significance of coronary topography of operative technique and tactics in multiple myocardial revascularization with jump grafts. Thorac Cardiovasc Surg 1981; 29:206–211.
6. Hutchins GM, Bulkley BH. Mechanisms of occlusion of saphenous vein-coronary artery "jump" graft. J Thorac Cardiovasc Surg 1977; 73:660–667.
7. Cheanvechai C, Groves LK, Surakiatchanukul S, Tanaka N, et al. Bridge saphenous vein graft. J Thorac Cardiovasc Surg 1975; 70:63–68.
8. Brower RW, van Eijk KF, Spek J, Bos E. Sequential versus conventional coronary artery bypass surgery in matched patient groups. Thorac Cardiovasc Surg 1981; 29:158–162.
9. Grondin CM, Limer R. Sequential anastomoses in coronary artery grafting: technical aspects and early and late angiographic results. Ann Thorac Surg 1976; 23:1–8.
10. Kieser TM, Fitzgibbon GM, Keon WJ. Sequential coronary bypass grafts. J Thorac Cardiovasc Surg 1986; 91:767–772.
11. Meurala H, Valle M, Hekaki P, Somer K, et al. Patency of sequential versus single vein grafts in coronary bypass surgery. Thorac Cardiovasc Surg 1982; 30:147–151.
12. Prioleau WH, Voegele LD, Hairston P. Flow in sequential vein grafts with diamond anastomosis. J Cardiovasc Surg 1986; 27:477–479.
13. O'Neill MJ Jr, Wolf PD, O'Neill TK, Montesano RM, et al. A rationale for the use of sequential coronary artery bypass grafts. J Thorac Cardiovasc Surg 1981; 81:686–690.

14. McNamara JJ, Bjerke HS, Chung GKT, Dang CR. Blood flow in sequential vein grafts. Circulation 1979; 60(2)suppl.:I–33–I–38.
15. Moreno-Cabral RJ, Mamuja RJ, Dang CR. Multiple coronary artery bypass using sequential technic. Am J Surg 1977; 134:64–69.
16. Yeh TJ, Heidary D, Shelton L. Y-grafts and sequential grafts in coronary bypass surgery: a critical evaluation of patency rates. Ann Thorac Surg 1979; 27(5):409–412.
17. Shioi K, Washizu T, Kawamura M, Abe T, et al. A study of sequential anastomosis in aortocoronary bypass surgery: internal configuration by the casting injection technique. Thorac Cardiovasc Surg 1984; 32:18–22.
18. Harjola PT, Meurala H, Jarvinen A. Sequential versus single aortocoronary saphenous vein bypass techniques. Ann Chir Gynaecol 1981; 70:191–196.
19. Minale C, Bourg NP, Bardos P, Messner BJ. Flow characteristics in single and sequential aorto-coronary bypass grafts. J Cardiovasc Surg 1984; 25:12–15.
20. Meester K, Veldkamp R, Tijssen JGP, van Herwerden LL, et al. Clinical outcome of single versus sequential grafts in coronary bypass operations at ten years follow-up. J Thorac Cardiovasc Surg 1991; 101:1076–1081.
21. Fujiwara T, Kajiya F, Kanazawa S, Matsuoha S, et al. Comparison of blood flow velocity waveforms in different coronary artery bypass grafts. Circulation 1988; 78:1210–1217.
22. Bigelow JC, Bartley TD, Page US, Krause AH. Long-term follow-up of sequential aortocoronary venous grafts. Ann Thorac Surg 1976; 22(16):507–514.
23. Crosby IK, Wellons HA Jr, Taylor GJ, Maffeo CJ, et al. Critical analysis of the preoperative and operative predictors of aortocoronary bypass patency. Ann Surg 1981; 193(6):743–751.
24. Loop FD, Lytle BS, Cosgrove DM. Influence of the internal-mammary-artery graft on 10 year survival and other events. N Engl J Med 1986; 314:1–6.

Chapter 18

The Innominate Artery-Coronary Artery Venous Bypass

Ronald K. Grooters and Hiroshi Nishida

The innominate artery-coronary artery venous bypass (ICVB) has been described[1,2] as a coronary grafting method used to avoid the embolic hazards of clamping a severely calcified aorta. Alternative methods of handling the diseased ascending aorta, such as occlusion of arch vessels with crossclamping and opening of the ascending aorta for inspection,[3] debridement of ascending aortic atherosclerosis,[4] or balloon catheter occlusion of the ascending aorta[5] have also been used successfully. Yet, these methods may risk embolization and a cerebral vascular accident because manipulation of the ascending aorta is still involved. The "no touch" technique described by Suma,[6] as well as bypass techniques that avoid instrumentation of the the ascending aorta, such as composite grafting (Chapter 15), subclavian-coronary artery grafting (Chapter 19), or a coronary-coronary artery bypass (Chapter 20) are also alternatives used for this challenging pathological condition. Whether or not a particular technique is used because of an atherosclerotic ascending aorta may depend on the surgeon's preference or the perceived feasibility of the situation. However, the ICVB is a possible alternative method of revascularization and needs to be part of the surgeon's armamentarium.

From Grooters RK and Nishida H: (editors): *Alternative Bypass Conduits and Methods for Surgical Coronary Revascularization.* © Futura Publishing Co., Inc., Armonk, NY, 1994.

Techniques

After the median sternotomy is made and the pericardium is opened, the ascending aorta should always be gently palpated. Once the ascending aorta is determined to be hazardous and the innominate artery is decided upon as a site for the proximal anastomosis, a site for arterial perfusion is picked. The femoral arteries are the first likely choices, but if both are occluded, a segment of healthy aorta beyond the takeoff of the innominate artery along the left lateral aspect of the aortic arch (Fig. 1) may accommodate cannulation. Once

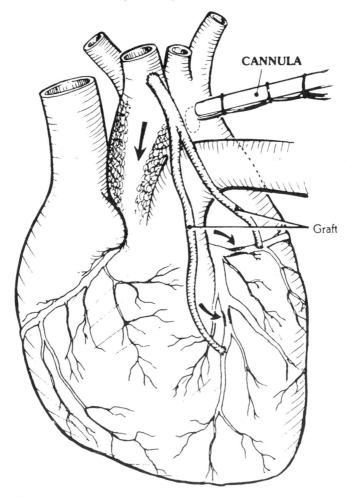

Fig. 1. The cannula site for arterial inflow is in the aortic arch at the base of the left common carotid artery (from Holland DL, et al.[2]).

cannulation is completed, cardiopulmonary bypass is instituted and the patient is cooled to 24°–28°C to protect the brain while the innominate artery is occluded during the construction of the ICVB. The hypothermia will also fibrillate the heart and allow the distal bypasses to be sutured. Ventricular venting may or may not be necessary. Although not clamping the ascending aorta is inconvenient and may not be as effective as cardioplegia techniques for preserving myocardium, excellent results are still possible.

Once the distal anastomoses are finished, the innominate artery is exposed by retracting cephalad the brachiocephalic vein. Vascular tapes or clamps are used to occlude the clean segment of the artery. If retracting the vein will not give exposure, it can be divided. The venous-innominate artery anastomosis is sutured with a continuous technique of 5-0 polypropylene. Before the clamps on the innominate artery are released, care must be taken to vent air or particulate debris by flushing the innominate artery prior to the completion of the anastomosis. The innominate artery occasionally may be large enough to accommodate a small side clamp that allows blood flow through the artery while the anastomosis is sutured. This allows rewarming of the patient after the distal grafts are completed, but if complete occlusion of the innominate artery is needed, the patient is not rewarmed until the anastomosis is nearly complete. A marker is placed around the anastomosis once it is finished, and the rest of the surgery is completed as usual.

Discussion

The type C severely atherosclerotic and calcified ascending aorta classified by Landymore et al.[7] definitely requires alternative methods of arterial perfusion (femoral, axillary, or aortic arch), continuous hypothermic coronary perfusion for myocardial preservation, and alternative placement of the proximal anastomosis. The ICVB can certainly be used in this situation, but occasionally the disease of the ascending aorta can involve the innominate artery as well. This may not be evident until manipulation or clamping of the artery. The innominate artery is prone to develop atherosclerosis and may even contain friable plaque or a stenosis without ascending aortic disease. We have observed these conditions with several postmortem examinations after unsuccessful bypass surgery.

We have also encountered disease in the innominate artery at the time of an ICVB grafting in a patient with an atherosclerotic ascending aorta. It was not until the vascular clamps were applied and the artery opened that the friable disease inside the artery was discovered. This patient sustained a right-sided hemispheric stroke but recovered.

This experience has influenced us to carefully consider ICVB grafting as well as other options for proximal graft sites such as (1) other arch vessels, (2) the internal mammary artery (IMA) pedicle as a site for the proximal anastomosis, or (3) the use of in situ arterial grafts with the "no touch" technique. Choosing one alternative instead of another may in part depend on the coronary anatomy and the conduits available. If three or more distal anastomoses are needed, liberal use of sequential grafting techniques can keep the number of proximal anastomoses to a minimum, preferably one. Weinstein and Killen[1] (Fig. 2) successfully used the sequential

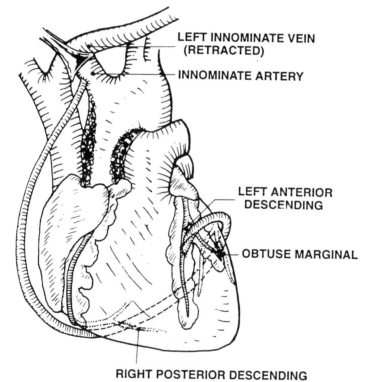

RIGHT POSTERIOR DESCENDING

Fig. 2. A sequential "snake" saphenous vein graft anastomosed to the anterior descending coronary artery (end-to-side) and then to the obtuse marginal and right posterior descending coronary arteries (side-to-side) with the proximal anastomosis snake to the innominate artery (from Weinstein G, et al.[1]).

"snake graft" technique, and Holland and Hieb[2] (Fig. 1) used in situ IMA grafting with venous Y grafts originating from the innominate artery. Although no large numbers of patients have been reported to facilitate a full review of this ICVB alternative, its use under certain circumstances is justifiable and should not be overlooked.

References

1. Weinstein G, Killen DA. Innominate artery-coronary artery bypass graft in a patient with calcific aortitis. J Thorac Cardiovasc Surg 1980; 79:312–313.
2. Holland DL, Hieb RE. Revascularization without embolization: coronary bypass in the presence of a calcified aorta. Ann Thorac Surg 1985; 40:308–310.
3. Landymore R, Spencer F, Colvin S, Culliford AT, et al. Management of the calcified aorta during myocardial revascularization. J Thorac Cardiovasc Surg 1982; 84:455–456.
4. Culliford AT, Colvin SB, Rohrer K, Baumann FG, et al. The atherosclerotic ascending aorta and transverse arch: a new technique to prevent cerebral injury during bypass: experience with 13 patients. Ann Thorac Surg 1986; 41:27–35.
5. Erath HG Jr, Stoney WS Jr. Balloon catheter occlusion of the ascending aorta. Ann Thorac Surg 1983; 35:560–561.
6. Suma H. Coronary artery bypass grafting in patients with calcified ascending aorta: aortic no-touch technique. Ann Thorac Surg 1989; 48:728–730.
7. Landymore R, Kinley CE. Classification and management of the diseased ascending aorta during cardiopulmonary bypass. J Thorac Cardiovasc Surg 1983; 85:639–640.

Chapter 19

The Subclavian Artery-Coronary Artery Venous Bypass

Ronald K. Grooters and Hiroshi Nishida

The subclavian artery-coronary artery venous bypass (SCAVB) has been reported to be very useful and effective in selected conditions for myocardial revascularization.[1–3] A left thoracotomy is the usual approach for this technique, but a median sternotomy, though not planned prior to the operation, has been used for this grafting.[4] Reoperations for coronary revascularization are becoming increasingly frequent, and, in some cases, reopening through a previous median sternotomy incision a second or third time can be hazardous and difficult. This is especially true if it is determined that a crossover internal mammary artery (IMA) grafting is patent or that previous grafts originate from an IMA pedicle or course directly behind the sternum. If a surgeon can anticipate that adequate or complete revascularization by means of an SCAVB will also produce a safer and easier operation in a patient with other preoperative conditions (i.e., a high- risk median sternotomy from previous multiple operations, previous mediastinitis, a diseased ascending aorta, concomitant left-chest pathology, or previous valve surgery), then this unique method of myocardial revascularization is a legitimate alternative.

Techniques

Most often, a left thoracotomy is used, and selective endotracheal intubation, though not mandatory, is very helpful with expo-

From Grooters RK and Nishida H: (editors): *Alternative Bypass Conduits and Methods for Surgical Coronary Revascularization.* © Futura Publishing Co., Inc., Armonk, NY, 1994.

sure (Fig. 1A). The patient is positioned for a left thoracotomy with the right leg exposed for a saphenous vein (SV) harvest. If the vein has been previously harvested, either the lesser SV or the left leg vein can be removed prior to positioning the patient. The patient's lower extremities and pelvis need to be rotated counterclockwise to the left to have the left femoral vessels available for cannulation. The chest is best entered through the fourth interspace, and resection of the fifth rib may be necessary to gain better exposure. Cardiopulmonary bypass (CPB) is not always necessary but should always be ready. If CPB is planned, cannulation for arterial perfusion can be done either using the femoral artery or descending aorta, and venous drainage can be accomplished with the left femoral vein or pulmonary artery

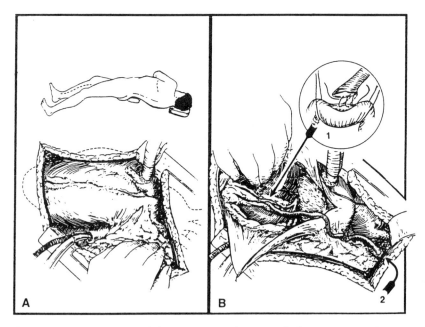

Fig. 1. (A) Positioning of the patient and pericardial incision used to approach the circumflex (CX) coronary artery using the left thoracotomy technique. (B) Saphenous vein (SV) bypass graft from the left subclavian artery to the circumflex system is performed by accomplishing the distal anastomosis (1) on the cold, fibrillating heart and then the proximal anastomosis (2) during the rewarming period (from Ungerleider RM, et al.[3]).

or both. If the descending aorta is severely atherosclerotic, the femoral artery usually is still satisfactory. The pulmonary artery is best cannulated with a right-angle venous cannula directed toward the pulmonary valve. If venous return is poor, additional venous drainage via the left femoral vein can be added. Usually, a size 32-to-36 cannula is more than adequate.

The pericardium is exposed and then opened posterior to the phrenic nerve. This is the best location if the circumflex system is to be grafted. Enough pericardial space is needed to place small defibrillatory paddles if fibrillation of the heart is needed. Once the patient is on CPB, the core temperature is dropped to 28°–30°C. The coronary artery to be bypassed is located and exposed during this period. A 2-0, or larger, ligature can be placed around the coronary artery, or, if exposure is challenging, myocardial sutures of the 2-0 or 3-0 size can be placed deep to the coronary artery for needed hemostatic control. The distal end of the graft is made ready for the anastomosis (Fig. 1B). A suture of 7-0 polypropylene is preferred. If the heart has not slowed appreciably, it is then fibrillated at this time. Gentle tension is then applied to the encircling sutures to control bleeding from the arteriotomy. If the heart is still too active or difficult to fibrillate, the body core temperature may be lowered to 22°C and blood flow reduced to approximately 1.0 L/min/m^2. We have not found it necessary to go any lower with the temperature or flow rate.

The anastomoses is then sutured with a continuous technique, and prior to finishing the suturing, rewarming is begun and the pump flow is increased. The proximal anastomosis is then constructed during the rewarming period using 5-0 or 6-0 polypropylene, usually to the left subclavian artery. A convenient or safe place without atherosclerosis on the descending aorta can also be used. A marker is placed around the proximal anastomosis for later identification if angiography is needed. When core body temperature (bladder or esophageal) reaches 36°C and the heart appears recovered, the patient is weaned from CPB. Two number 36 chest tubes are inserted and fixed with heavy silk suture, and the thoracotomy is closed.

If the median sternotomy approach is used, the subclavian vessels can be approached anteriorly. We have found that a "hockey-stick" extension of the median sternotomy directed superiorly to the side of the subclavian artery to be grafted will facilitate exposure for suturing the anastomosis.

Descending Aorta-Coronary Artery Venous Bypass

A convenient or safe place (without atherosclerosis) on the descending aorta is also appropriate. We recently used the left thoracotomy approach to bypass a stenotic large circumflex (CX) coronary artery with unstable angina on medical therapy. The cardiologists involved were reluctant, unbelievably, to dilate the lesion because of its size and an associated tight left main stenosis (Fig. 2A). The patient had undergone a three-vessel vein bypass to the diagonal coronary artery, left anterior descending (LAD) artery, and posterior descending (PD) artery concomitant with a Y graft from the ascending aorta to both common carotid arteries 4 years previously. The Dacron Y graft was suspected to be adherent to the sternum, and little or no room was left on the ascending aorta for other grafting or crossclamp placement. The technique just described was used but, at the time of surgery, the proximal left subclavian vessel was found to be severely atherosclerotic. Normal descending aorta located 4–5 cm below the origin of the left subclavian was identified, side-clamped, and used as the site of the proximal anastomosis. The path of the graft, when finished, was posterior and inferior to the hilum of the left lung and followed a parallel course with the descending aorta until it angled medially to the CX. Angiography 10 days after surgery revealed a patent graft, and the patient has remained asymptomatic (Fig. 2B).

Discussion

The SCAVB is a unique grafting method generally used to avoid certain potentially dangerous operative situations in patients requiring myocardial revascularization to the LAD or CX. The left thoracotomy for an SCAVB grafting is the usual approach (Fig. 1). Appropriate examples are patients with patent grafts, an ascending aorta likely to be adherent beneath the sternum, or a history of previous valve surgery. Left lung pathology, particularly on the left lower lobe (because it is inaccessible from a median sternotomy) with concomitant left coronary artery pathology is another combination amenable to an SCAVB.[2,3] We have also used this method of grafting for a patient with an acute descending aortic dissection and a significant stenosis of a large CX. The dissection, which had spared the left subclavian artery and the ascending aorta, was repaired first with a

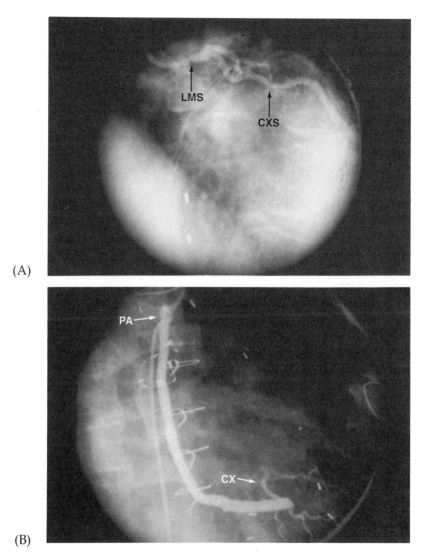

Fig. 2. (A) Angiogram of a patient with left main stenosis and a stenosis of a larger circumflex in a patient with previous bypass surgery and a sternotomy infection. LMS:left main stenosis; CXS: circumflex stenosis. (B) Angiogram of the descending aorta-circumflex vein graft. PA: proximal anastomosis. Right anterior oblique view.

Dacron tube graft. Because this part of the operation went very well, we proceeded on to the CX grafting using the SCAVB grafting. The patient recovered nicely and was discharged on the tenth postoperative day. A treadmill test 2 months later was normal. We were quite sure that this patient would have suffered a major cardiac event if the coronary stenosis had been ignored. Additionally, we prevented any later postoperative coronary intervention.

The SCAVB grafting can also be done via a median sternotomy (Fig. 3). Bilgutay and colleagues[4] used this grafting method from the left subclavian artery in one patient with an ascending aortic dissec-

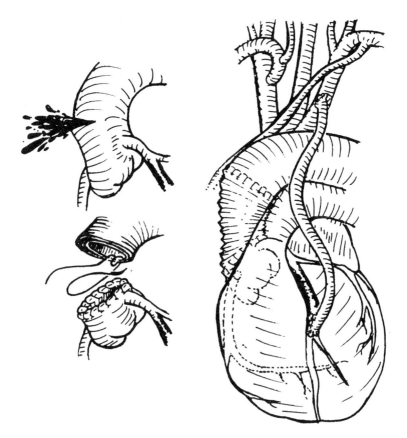

Fig. 3. Completion of repair of a dissection with the interposition of a woven Teflon graft and a left-subclavian-to-left-anterior-descending coronary artery vein bypass (from Bilgutay AM, et al.[4]).

tion, which happened shortly after CPB using femoral cannulation. This same group[4] also used a right SCAVB to the right PD in another patient with a spontaneous dissection limited to the ascending aorta (Fig. 4). Before the right or left subclavian artery is used as the origin of a vein graft, the innominate artery first needs to be considered as an alternative method of coronary grafting (Chapter 18). Any pathology involving the innominate artery, such as dissection or atherosclerosis, may preclude the right subclavian artery as the origin of the vein graft. Other sites for a proximal anastomosis, such as an IMA composite graft (Chapter 15), or a coronary-coronary artery bypass

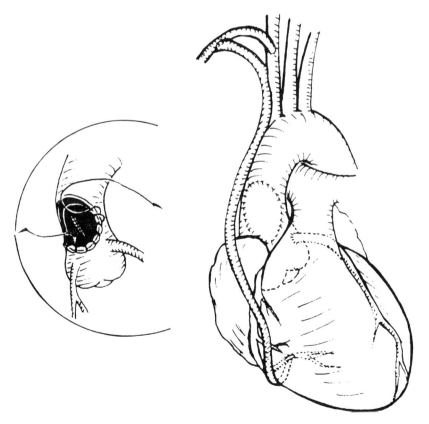

Fig. 4. Diagrammatic representation in a case of patch repair of an ascending dissection and a right-subclavian-to-right-coronary-artery saphenous vein bypass (from Bilgutay AM, et al.[4]).

(Chapter 20), or grafts originating from a patch of the ascending aorta (Chapter 23, Fig. 6) are also appropriate alternatives to consider in the situation described by Bilgutay et al.[4]

References

1. Aquom AS, Ray JF III, Sanoudos GM, Moollem S, et al. Subclavian-coronary artery bypass in man. J Thorac Cardiovasc Surg 1973; 65(6): 869–871.
2. Faro RS, Javid H, Najafi H, Serry C. Left thoracotomy for reoperation for coronary revascularization. J Thorac Cardiovasc Surg 1982; 84:453–455.
3. Ungerleider RM, Mills NL, Wechsler AS. Left thoracotomy for reoperative coronary artery bypass procedures. Ann Thorac Surg 1985; 40:11–15.
4. Bilgutay AM, Garamella JT, Danyluk M, Ramucal HC. Retrograde aortic dissection occurring during cardiopulmonary bypass: successful repair on concomitant subclavian-to-coronary artery vein bypass. JAMA 1976; 236(5):465–468.

Chapter 20

The Coronary-Coronary Bypass Graft

Hiroshi Nishida, Masahiro Endo, and
Hitoshi Koyanagi

Coronary artery to coronary artery bypass grafting (CCBG) using the saphenous vein (SV) was first introduced in 1987 by Rowland
and Grooters.[1] This technique was applied successfully to a patient
with calcification of the ascending aorta that was unsuitable for the
conventional saphenous vein aortocoronary bypass graft (ACBG)
(Fig. 1) and to a patient with an inadequate length of graft. In 1989,
Nishida and associates[2] reported the first CCBG using the free right
internal thoracic artery (ITA) to bypass the distal posterior descending (PD) artery with the proximal anastomosis on the right coronary
artery (RCA) (Fig. 2) in a patient who had no vein conduit. During
this same period of time, Biglioli and colleagues[3] postulated that this
technique takes advantage of the physiological position of the right
coronary ostium, which originates from the sinus of Valsalva. They
also postulated that filling of the proximal coronary artery is, in
part, promoted by the protodiastolic inversion of blood flow in the
ascending aorta and the consequent distension of the sinuses, thus
acting as a reservoir keeping diastolic flow constant to the coronary
artery graft.

Clinical Experience

We have performed CCBG in 29 patients with no mortality (Table
1). The graft patency confirmed with angiography was 96.7%.

From Grooters RK and Nishida H: (editors): *Alternative Bypass Conduits and Methods for
Surgical Coronary Revascularization.* © Futura Publishing Co., Inc., Armonk, NY, 1994.

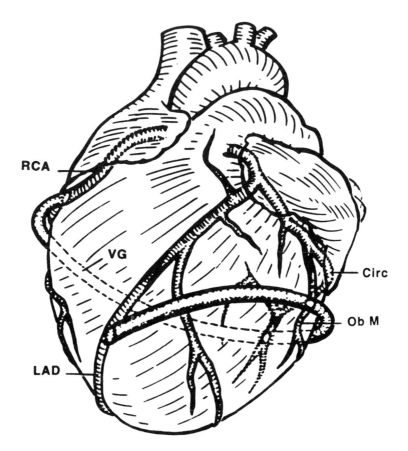

Fig. 1. Left anterior oblique projection demonstrating a sequential vein graft (VG) between the right coronary artery (RCA), circumflex artery (Circ), obtuse marginal (Obm), and left anterior descending artery (LAD) (from Rowland RE, et al.[1]).

Twenty-six patients underwent CCBG within the same coronary artery (intracoronary CCBG), in which the proximal coronary artery was used as a donor artery to the distal segment of the same coronary artery, such as a CCBG from the RCA to the PD. The other three patients underwent intercoronary artery type CCBG, in which the proximal part of a coronary artery was used as the donor artery distally to a different coronary artery. In five cases, the CCBG was established as a sequential bypass with two distal anastomoses (CC sequential bypass).

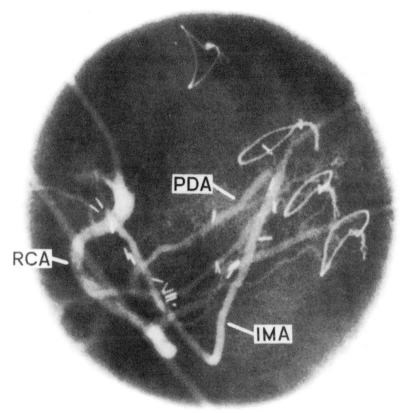

Fig. 2. The coronary-coronary artery bypass using right free internal mammary (IMA) between the proximal right coronary artery (RCA) and posterior descending artery (PDA). (from Nishida H, et al.[2]).

Because of the initial success of this technique, other free arterial grafts such as the right gastroepiploic artery (RGEA) and the inferior epigastric artery (IEA) have been used in this manner. This technique increases the distance to which a free arterial graft can be used to bypass distal coronary arteries, thus providing more of an opportunity for a complete revascularization with arterial grafts. In addition, we have found that construction of the proximal anastomosis of a free arterial graft to a normal proximal coronary artery is easier and simpler than directly placing it on the aorta, to a hood of SV,[4] to a patch of SV,[5] or a pericardial aortic patch.[6] The IEA can be used only as a

Table 1
**Coronary-Coronary Bypass Graft
(1987–1992)**

Total No. of Patients:	29 cases
Gender:	25 males
	4 females
Age:	49–72 (59.6 ± 7.1) yrs
No. of Diseased Vessels:	1 single
	2 double
	18 triple
	8 LMT
No. of Bypasses:	1–5 (2.9 ± 0.8/patient)
Bypass Conduit:	21 SV
	4 RITA
	1 LITA
	1 RGEA
	2 IEA
Early Results:	0 operative deaths
	0 hospital deaths
	0 perioperative infarctions
	44.5 ± 36.0 mL/min graft flow
	96.6% (28/29) patency

LMT: left main trunk; RITA: right internal thoracic artery; LITA: left internal thoracic artery

free graft; therefore, a coronary-to-coronary graft can be an important alternative method to be used with this conduit (Fig. 3).

Experimental Work

To compare flow in the CCBG with that in the ACBG to the same coronary bed and to determine the flow reserve of the proximal RCA as a donor vessel to the CCBG, we performed the experiment in eight mongrel dogs.[7] Both a CCBG and ACBG were constructed to the proximally ligated left anterior descending artery (LAD). The flow of each graft was measured with the other graft temporarily occluded (Fig. 4). RCA flow proximal to the anastomosis (average internal diameter 1.5 mm) was measured before and after the opening of the CCBG (Fig. 5). This flow of the proximal RCA increased from 35.4 ± 11.8 mL/min to 76.0 ± 15.3 mL/min after opening the CCBG, which had a flow rate of 42.2 ± 10.4 mL/min. The flow of the ACBG was compared to the CCBG flow, and no difference was found (Fig. 6).

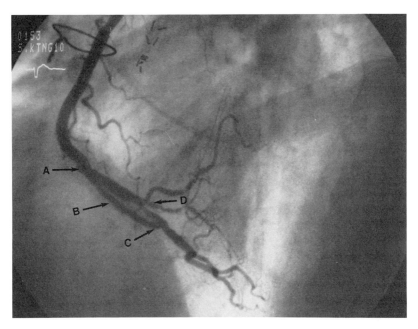

Fig. 3. The use of the inferior epigastric artery (IEA) to bypass from the right coronary artery (RCA) distal to the posterior descending artery (PD). A—proximal anastomosis; B—inferior epigastric artery graft; C—distal anastomosis; D—RCA stenosis.

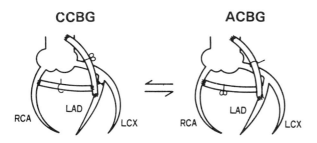

Fig. 4. Flow in the coronary-coronary bypass graft (CCBG) and aortocoronary bypass graft (ACBG) was measured independently while the other graft was temporarily occluded (from Nishida H, et al.[7]).

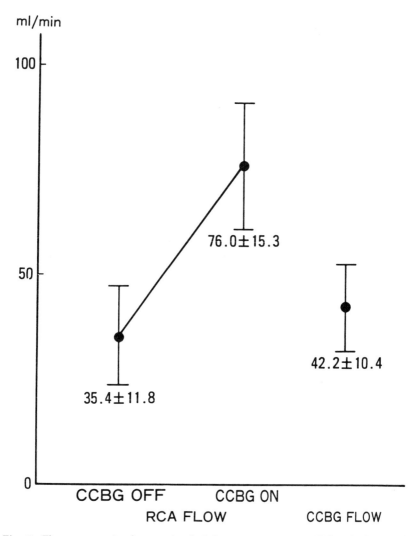

Fig. 5. Flow reserve in the proximal right coronary artery (RCA) before and after opening the coronary-coronary bypass graft (CCBG) (from Nishida H, et al.[7]).

Flow curve studies also demonstrated early systolic flow reversal in the ACBG, while the CCBG showed only forward flow (Fig. 7). We believe that this difference is related to different origins of the ACBG and CCBG. The ACBG originates from the ascending aorta distal to

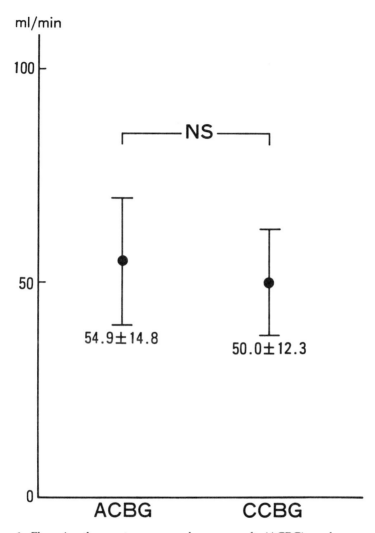

Fig. 6. Flow in the aortocoronary bypass graft (ACBG) and coronary-coronary bypass graft (CCBG) (from Nishida H, et al.[7]).

the sinus of Valsalva, whereas the CCBG originates from the native coronary artery, which itself arises from the sinus of Valsalva. We conclude from this study that the CCBG can provide nearly the same flow rate as the ACBG and that the proximal RCA has sufficient flow reserve for this technique.

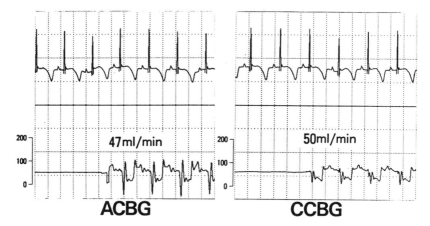

Fig. 7. Flow curves showing early systolic flow reversal in aortocoronary bypass graft (ACBG) and forward flow only in the coronary-coronary bypass graft (CCBG) (from Nishida H, et al.[7]).

Technical Aspects of the Coronary-Coronary Bypass Graft

The proximal coronary artery used to feed the graft should be large and free of disease. The placement of the feeding anastomosis should be as proximal as possible to provide maximal flow reserve capacity, even though the flow and patency of the graft also depends on distal runoff of the coronary artery and the size of the graft. Therefore, the graft should be at least the diameter of the coronary artery, especially if the smaller diameter arterial grafts are used. We feel that the internal thoracic artery is the ideal graft conduit because of its size, as well as the excellent patency rate.

The proximal anastomosis is most easily constructed or sometimes can only be constructed during the crossclamp period. This will then prolong the ischemic time for the myocardium by 10 to 15 minutes, but this has not increased the perioperative infarction rate or the mortality rate. If the ascending aorta is severely diseased, prohibiting aortic crossclamping or side-clamping, the proximal coronary can be occluded with a bulldog clamp. This is most easily done on the RCA since exposure is quite easy.

Conclusion

This alternative method may assist the surgeon with the three major problems we face today in surgical coronary artery revascularizations: (1) a shortage of graft material caused by increased number of reoperations; (2) an increased number of perioperative strokes resulting from the severely atheromatous or calcified aorta seen more frequently in older patients; and (3) the expanding demand for complete revascularization with arterial grafts, which are limited in amount and length.

References

1. Rowland RE, Grooters RK. Coronary-coronary artery bypass: an alternative. Ann Thorac Surg 1987: 43:326–328.
2. Nishida H, Soltanzadeh H, Grooters RK, Thieman KC. Coronary-coronary bypass with internal mammary artery. Ann Thorac Surg 1988; 46:577–578.
3. Biglioli P, Alamanni F, Antona C, Sala A, et al. Coronary-coronary bypass: theoretical basis and techniques. J Cardiovasc Surg 1987; 28:333–335.
4. Barner HB. The internal mammary artery as a free graft. J Thorac Cardiovasc Surg 1973; 66:219–221.
5. Schimert G, Vinde B, Lee AB Jr. Free internal mammary artery graft: an improved surgical technique. Ann Thorac Surg 1975; 19:474–477.
6. Kanter KR, Barner HB. Improved technique for the proximal anastomosis with free internal mammary artery grafts. Ann Thorac Surg 1987; 44:556–557.
7. Nishida H, Grooters RK, Endo M, Koyanagi H, et al. Flow study of coronary-coronary bypass graft. Cardiovasc Surg 1993; 1:296–299.

Chapter 21

The Selective Retrograde Coronary Venous Bypass

Ronald K. Grooters and Hiroshi Nishida

In the early 1970s, cardiovascular surgeons were confronted with extensive and diffuse atherosclerotic disease of one or more coronary arteries that could not be successfully bypassed. This patient group represented 12%–15% of possible candidates for revascularization.[1] In order to benefit these unfortunate patients, the selective retrograde coronary venous bypass (SRCVB) was investigated and performed clinically by a number of investigators.[2–9]

In 1889, Pratt[10] had postulated the possibility of retrovenous coronary perfusion and suggested that the heart could be effectively nourished by retrograde perfusion through the coronary sinus or thebesius vessels. By 1930, Batson and Bellet[11] found that when the pressure in the capillary bed is low from the occlusion of two coronary arteries, flow in the vein during atrial systole is probably toward the capillary bed, which then empties during the ensuing ventricular systole. Beck et al.,[12] in 1948, reported the method of a systemic artery-coronary sinus anastomosis (the Beck II procedure), which included a partial occlusion of the coronary sinus toward the right atrium done at a second operation. The mortality was high (29%), and the procedure was eventually abandoned. Bakst and Bailey[13] did demonstrate with this procedure that (1) retrograde perfusion of the myocardium does occur, (2) myocardial extraction of oxygen during retrograde perfusion is measurable, and (3) increased intercoronary

From Grooters RK and Nishida H: (editors): *Alternative Bypass Conduits and Methods for Surgical Coronary Revascularization.* © Futura Publishing Co., Inc., Armonk, NY, 1994.

collateral flow is present. This study also demonstrated obliterative changes in the coronary vein (CV) within a few weeks of the operation.

Arealis and colleagues[2] were the first to demonstrate experimentally the potential immediate beneficial effects of myocardial perfusion by anastomosing the internal mammary artery (IMA) to a ligated coronary vein. Other surgeons[6-8] demonstrated in dog studies that frequently the myocardium became stiffened and hemorrhagic. Additionally, the survivors at 3 to 6 weeks developed progressive CV obliterative change. Other surgeons[3,4,9] did not observe these detrimental changes but postulated that the IMA flow might be inadequate. In their studies, the conclusions were made that the flow in the graft to the CV should be 50 mL/min or greater and that a vein graft may provide the needed improved flow. A few clinical short-term successes were obtained by Park et al.,[3] Benedict et al.,[4] and Moll et al.,[5] but soon the procedure lost favor as a result of alternative arterial revascularization techniques such as sequential grafting, coronary artery patching techniques, and extensive coronary endarterectomy. The last extensive research reported on the SRCVB technique (Fig. 1) was by Hockberg and colleagues[14] in 1979, which demonstrated effective perfusion of all layers of the myocardium using the SRCVB. They also concluded that encouraging long-term patency data in animals (3 to 5 months) suggested that possible judicious use of this bypass method might be of value in selected patients with diffuse atherosclerosis or a previously failed coronary artery bypass. Did we abandon this technique too soon?

Experimental Studies

Arealis and colleagues,[2] at the University of Utah, first proposed the SRCVB using an IMA to bypass a ligated left anterior descending vein (LADV). In calves, they demonstrated reversal of electrocardiographic (ECG) changes caused by ligating the left anterior descending artery (LAD). A year later, Bhayana and colleagues,[15] at the same institution, confirmed, using sheep, the reversibility of ischemic ST segment ECG changes following construction of the IMA bypass to the LADV. Flow rates ranged from 20–90 cc/min. Perfusion of the vein was stopped after 60 minutes while the LAD remained occluded. ST segment changes indicative of ischemia then returned. Park and coworkers[3] demonstrated, using dogs, that 20% of the blood

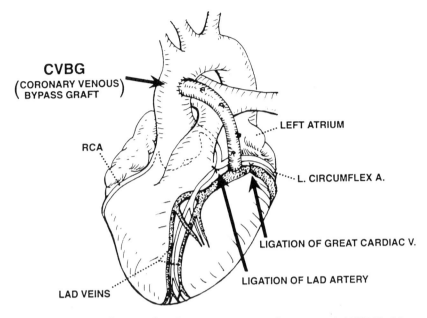

Fig. 1. Diagram of a completed coronary venous bypass graft (CVBG). Note proximal ligation of the LAD artery to render the anterior wall ischemic. The LAD vein was also ligated cephalad to the CVBG to prevent an arteriovenous fistula (from Hockberg MS, et al.[14]).

flow from an IMA-SRCVB reached the coronary sinus as a direct shunt; they concluded that 80% of the flow was available for oxygen extraction from the myocardium. Additionally, they felt that the IMA-SRCVB did not prevent infarction if the LAD was closed abruptly, but when the LAD was occluded gradually with an ameroid constrictor, reverse myocardial perfusion was able to function, and myocardial infarction did not occur. Demos and colleagues[16] reported, using pigs, that maintaining SRCVB flow rates of 40–60 mL/min prevented ECG ischemic changes after LAD ligation. Also, interstitial hemorrhage and infarction did not occur over the short term of the experiment (3 hours).

Chiu and Mulder[17] investigated the IMA-SRCVB after the LAD occlusion in sheep. Flow rates to the CV were 50–200 mL/min. When put to death 10 days to 5 months after operation, no evidence of edema or hemorrhage was found, and mature infarcts were smaller in the graft group versus the control group in whom no grafts were performed after LAD ligation. Corrosion casts also demonstrated patency of the venous tree as well as veno-venous collateral runoff channels. Benedict et al.[4] compared IMA and free femoral vein usage for the SRCVB in dogs. Using an electromagnetic flow meter, radioisotope scanning, methylene blue injections, a coronary angiogram, and a hydrogen electrode evaluation of arteriovenous shunting and venous capillary response to papaverine and isoproterenol, the IMA inflow was frequently less than 50 mL/min and thus a poor method of retrograde coronary venous perfusion. The SV provided better flow rates and protection. Myocardial hemorrhage and infarction occurred only after the third attempt at major ligation of draining venous collaterals.

Not all investigators demonstrated favorable results. Kay and Suzuki[6] performed IMA-SRCVBs in dogs, and they noted reversal of myocardial ischemia during the first hour following myocardial hemorrhage and stiffening. However, these changes were reversed by grafting the LAD to the left atrium to shunt off excess congestion. Zajtchuk and associates[7] found that the protection provided by the IMA-SRCVB was of short duration and also found severe intimal stenosis of the CV in the survivors at 6 to 8 months postoperatively. Marco and colleagues[8] demonstrated short-term benefit in dogs from the IMA-SRCVB, with a mortality rate at 6 weeks of only 14% in the grafted group as compared to a 40% mortality rate for the ungrafted control group. Angiography at 6 weeks demonstrated IMA patency, but the recipient veins demonstrated severe obliterative changes. Postmortem examination showed intimal proliferation, subintimal fibrosis, and medial hypertrophy. These investigators concluded that the SRCVB provided only short-term benefit, and long-term progression of cardiac vein obliteration limited its use in humans to only desperate situations.

In the last reported extensive research by Hockberg and colleagues,[14] favorable results were obtained. Using dogs to evaluate SRCVB long-term (3 to 5 months) effectiveness, 10 out of 14 grafts were patent angiographically. Transmural flow was 39 ± 1 mL per 100 grams of tissue per minute. Flow to all layers of the myocardium was confirmed by utilizing microsphere flow measurements developed by Rudolph and Heymann.[18] Histologic examination found no evidence of venous sclerosis or thrombosis and no evidence of myocardial interstitial edema or hemorrhage. This animal study suggested that judicious use of a venous bypass could be of value in selected patients.

Clinical Experience

Three reports on the clinical usage of SRCVB appear in the literature. Benedict and colleagues[4] used saphenous vein (SV) grafts to the LADV in three patients with intractable angina pectoris and previous unsuccessful revascularization procedures. All three patients survived and, when myocardial scanning was used, demonstrated adequate perfusion of the myocardial segments served by the patent grafts. Angiography of two patients revealed two patent grafts, and the third patient felt so good that he refused restudy. These authors also suggested that the epicardium be incorporated into the suture line because the veins were so thin. They also determined that no more than two major veins should be grafted to ensure pathways for coronary venous return. Park and associates[3] performed the SRCVB with an IMA in six patients with diffuse atherosclerosis with poor or no runoff of the LAD. All of the patients had satisfactory left ventricular contraction. Concomitant vein grafts were constructed to bypassable coronary arteries. The six patients were free of angina at 1 year. Follow-up angiography in three patients at 2 ½–7 months postsurgery revealed one graft occluded, one graft patent but with a predominant arteriovenous shunt and little myocardial uptake demonstrated during a scan, and another graft patent with excellent myocardial uptake on scanning.

The largest clinical application of SRCVB was reported by Moll and coworkers.[5] Twenty-one patients with diffuse peripheral atherosclerotic disease of the distal coronary arteries, five of whom had preoperative cardiogenic shock, received at least one SRCVB. Fifteen patients survived. Five deaths were from the cardiogenic shock group, and one other patient died 3 months after surgery as a result of circulatory failure due to cardiac aneurysm and cerebral embolism. The 15 surviving patients showed good immediate clinical and ECG findings. The authors concluded that the early results were very encouraging, but that long-term observation was needed to assess the behavior of the arterialized veins subject to high pressure. Unfortunately, no long-term follow-up studies were reported.

Discussion

It is intriguing that the last major research effort by Hockberg and colleagues[14] seems to show a possible positive place for the SRCVB, yet no further studies, animal or clinical, have since been reported. These surgeons also provided a rationale for the discrepancy in findings between investigators[7,8] who reported little or no benefit from the SRCVB and those SRCVB researchers[2–4,15–17] who demonstrated encouraging experiments. First, the IMA inflow may have been inadequate. Zajtchuk's group[7] and Marco's study[8] did not measure SRCVB flow at the time of operation, and this may have accounted for their dismal results. Second, the point of LAD ligation may have been different in these studies. Fatal arterial infarction in dogs can be achieved only if the artery is occluded proximal to the first septal perforator. With ligation distal to this branch, arterial inflow via this perforator and collaterals may be competitive and cause the IMA-CV inflow to be far less significant at the capillary level, thus increasing the possibility of a higher closure rate. This could well be the cause for failure of the IMA-LADV anastomoses in the study by Marco.[8] A third discrepancy may be the metabolic sampling from the coronary sinus. As suggested by Hammond and Austen,[19] greater than 50% of LAD blood flow is returned to the heart by routes other than the coronary sinus. Reports of retrograde perfusion based on coronary sinus sampling may not always be reflective of myocardial perfusion. Fourth, the papers not supportive of SRCVB reported that the anastomoses were achieved without cardiopulmonary bypass. Hockberg et al.[14] state that they found that a more precise anastomosis could be constructed with a quiet heart.

Are these differences enough of an explanation and, if so, should we accept the encouraging results of the latest research effort?[14] We know that some clinical success[3–5] had been obtained, yet from what was reported, no significant long-term conclusion could be made. It may very well be reasonable to offer this alternative to the desperate patient with diffuse atherosclerosis (not amenable to endarterectomy or transplantation) or to patients in whom multiple conventional coronary artery bypass procedures have acutely failed.

References

1. Bates RJ, Toscano M, Balderman SC, Anagnostipoulous CE. The cardiac veins and retrograde coronary venous perfusion. Ann Thorac Surg 1977; 23:83–90.
2. Arealis EG, Volder JGR, Kolff WJ. Arterialization of the coronary vein coming from an ischemic area. Chest 1973; 63:462–463.
3. Park SB, Magovern GJ, Liebler GA, Dixon CM, et al. Direct selective myocardial revascularization by internal mammary artery-coronary vein anastomosis. J Thorac Cardiovasc Surg 1975; 69:63–72.

4. Benedict JS, Buhl TL, Henney RP. Cardiac vein myocardial revascularization. Ann Thorac Surg 1975; 20:550–557.
5. Moll JW, Dziatkowiak AJ, Edelman M, Iljin W, et al. Arterialization of the coronary veins in diffuse coronary atherosclerosis. J Cardiovasc Surg 1975; 16:520–525.
6. Kay EB, Suzuki A. Coronary venous retroperfusion for myocardial revascularization. Ann Thorac Surg 1975; 19:327–330.
7. Zajtchuk R, Heydorn WH, Miller JG, Strevey TE, et al. Revascularization of the heart through the coronary veins. Ann Thorac Surg 1976; 21:318–321.
8. Marco JD, Hahn JW, Barner HB, Jellinek M, et al. Coronary venous arterialization: acute hemodynamic, metabolic, and chronic anatomical observations. Ann Thorac Surg 1977; 23:449–454.
9. Hockberg MS. Hemodynamic evaluation of selective arterialization of the coronary venous system. J Thorac Cardiovasc Surg 1977; 74:774–783.
10. Pratt FH. The nutrition of the heart through the vessels of thebesius and the coronary veins. Am J Physiol 1889; 1:86–89.
11. Batson OV, Bellet S. The reversal of flow in cardiac veins. Am Heart J 1930; 6:206–209.
12. Beck CS, Stanton E, Batilechuk W. Revascularization of heart by graft of systemic artery into coronary sinus. JAMA 1948; 137:436–442.
13. Bakst AA, Bailey CP. Arterialization of the coronary sinus in occlusive coronary artery disease: IV. Coronary flow in dogs with aortocoronary sinus anastomosis of twelve months duration. J Thorac Surg 1956; 31:559–568.
14. Hockberg MS, Roberts WC, Morrow AG, Austen WG. Selective arterialization of the coronary venous system. J Thorac Cardiovasc Surg 1979; 77:1–12.
15. Bhayana JW, Olsen DB, Byrne JP, Kolff WJ. Reversal of myocardial ischemia by arterialization of the coronary vein. J Thorac Cardiovasc Surg 1974; 67(1):125–132.
16. Demos S, Brooks H, Holland R, Balderman S, et al. Retrograde coronary venous perfusion to reverse and prevent acute myocardial ischemia. Circulation 1974; 49(suppl.3):168.
17. Chiu CJ, Mulder OS. Selective arterialization of coronary veins for diffuse coronary occlusion: an experimental evaluation. J Thorac Cardiovasc Surg 1975; 70:177–182.
18. Rudolph AM, Heymann MA. The circulation of the fetus in utero: methods for studying distribution of blood flow, cardiac output, and organ blood flow. Circ Res 1967; 21:163–184.
19. Hammond GL, Austen WG. Drainage patterns of coronary arterial flow as determined from the isolated heart. Am J Physiol 1967; 212:1435–1440.

Chapter 22

Sequential Vein Coronary Artery Grafting With a Surgical Atrial Fistula

Hiroshi Nishida, Masahiro Endo,
Hitoshi Koyanagi, and Ronald K. Grooters

Sequential bypass grafting has been and still is a widely used alternative method of coronary artery revascularization,[1,2] which has the advantages of preserving conduit and increasing the total conduit blood flow and results in a potentially higher graft patency (Chapter 17). This technique may be especially advantageous in situations of extremely poor coronary runoff due to multiple small or diffusely diseased vessels. An ideal combination of obstructed coronary arteries even for sequential techniques does not always exist, particularly if a situation is encountered in which total graft flow may not be sufficient to ensure good graft patency. If this problem can be anticipated, a surgical fistula using the distal end of the conduit as the last anastomosis constructed to a low-pressure cardiac chamber (right or left atrium) may increase graft flow and improve patency. A similar concept of surgical arteriovenous fistulization has been successfully applied during the revascularization of ischemic extremities.[3,4] Recently, this method has been successful using a "snake graft" technique during coronary artery revascularization by fistulizing the end of the graft to the right atrium.[5]

From Grooters RK and Nishida H: (editors): *Alternative Bypass Conduits and Methods for Surgical Coronary Revascularization.* © Futura Publishing Co., Inc., Armonk, NY, 1994.

Clinical Experience

In 1988, Spampinato and colleagues[5] reported on four patients who received a sequential bypass. The surgeons made three to four side-to-side anastomoses to diseased coronary arteries, with the last anastomosis sutured to the right atrium, creating an intentional surgical coronary artery vein graft-atrial fistula. The left anterior descending (LAD) artery was the target vessel for the last sequential anastomosis, but in three of the four patients the LAD was small. The determination was made that the LAD in each of these patients did not provide adequate runoff to improve the total graft flow of the long sequential bypass and that patency might be jeopardized. Therefore, the anastomosis to the LAD was performed side-to-side, and the remaining segment of the vein graft was anastomosed to the right atrium (Fig. 1). The last anastomosis was calibrated by progressively tightening the purse string of the atrial suture, while the flow through the graft was measured with a magnetic flowmeter to achieve the desired flow rate. This final accepted flow rate was not reported. There were no operative deaths, and all patients experienced clinical improvement. No adverse hemodynamics were observed in the postoperative period. Two patients underwent coronary angiography 6 and 8 months after surgery. All anastomoses were patent, plus a small "puff" of dye into the right atrium was seen (Fig. 2). No steal flow from the coronary artery system was observed angiographically.

Experimental Work

We conducted an experimental study to measure graft flow, assess cardiac hemodynamics, determine graft flow distribution, and also determine the proper size of the distal anastomosis (DA), the fistula. A saphenous vein (SV) was sequentially anastomosed from the ascending aorta to the LAD, and the distal anastomosis (DA) was constructed to the left atrial appendage (LA) in eight mongrel dogs (Fig. 3). The LAD was proximally ligated. Graft flow (mL/min) was measured between the aorta and LAD (flow no. 1) and between the LAD and LA (flow no. 2) before and after opening the fistula to the LA. Flow no. 1 is the total graft flow with flow no. 2 (the shunt flow) open to the LA. Flow no. 1 minus flow no. 2 reflects the flow to the LAD. When the fistula is closed, flow no. 1 becomes the flow to the

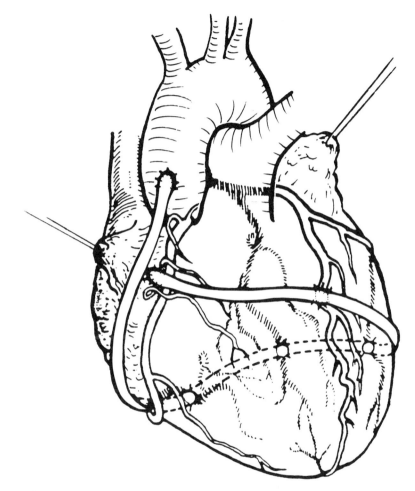

Fig. 1. Drawing of the technique employed (from Spampinato N, et al.[5]).

LAD, and flow no. 2 is zero. Left atrial pressure (LAP) and systolic left ventricular pressure (LVP) (mm Hg) were recorded. The DA diameter was regulated using a bulldog clamp and measured with calipers. When the DA was 2.5 to 3 mm in diameter, flow no. 1 increased from 64.5 + 19.5 to 134.7 + 28.5 ($p < 0.01$) (Fig. 4), without significant LAP or LVP change (Fig. 5). In contrast, when the DA was 4 mm

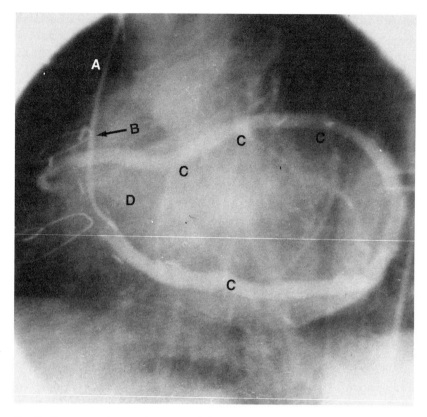

Fig. 2. Postoperative angiogram in left anterior oblique showing the patency of the graft and the anastomoses. The catheter is well inside the vein graft almost at the level of the acute margin of the heart. A: aortic anastomosis; B: catheter pushed inside the graft almost to the acute margin of the heart; C: the grafts; D: dye puff into the right atrium (from Spampinato N, et al.[5]).

or more, flow no. 1 increased from $69.8 + 1.0$ to $396.1 + 62.2$ ($p < 0.001$). LAP increased from $5.6 + 1.0$ to $6.1 + 0.9$ ($p < 0.05$) without a significant change in LVP. Figure 6 demonstrates the increments of total flow volume and, with the increase in the size of the fistula, flow rates to the LAD remain stable.

The pattern of shunt flow to the LA flow no. 2 was mainly systolic. The pattern of flow no. 1 was diastolic dominant before opening

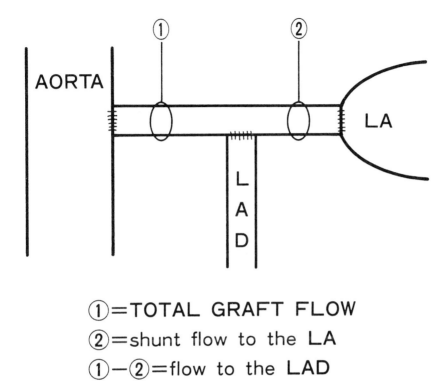

①=TOTAL GRAFT FLOW

②=shunt flow to the LA

①−②=flow to the LAD

Fig. 3. Schematic explanation and definition of flow measurement.

the fistula but changed to biphasic flow superimposing the systolic dominant flow (flow no. 2). With the different sizes of the DA, flow to the LAD did not change either before or after the fistula was opened. This indicated no steal phenomenon, even with a large amount of shunt flow from the aorta to the LA (Fig. 6). Volume loading, rapid atrial pacing, and neosynephrine or epinephrine infusions caused no deleterious hemodynamic effects when the fistula was open to any size. In conclusion, a surgical coronary artery fistulization of 2.5 to 3 mm in diameter will effectively increase total graft flow without decreasing flow to the bypassed coronary artery and will not cause significant deleterious cardiac hemodynamics such as volume overload of the left ventricle. Flows of 350 to 450 cc/min through the fistula are also well tolerated.

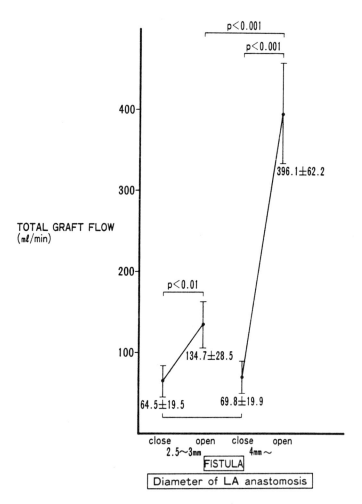

Fig. 4. Total graft flow depends on the size of the fistula and increases significantly when the diameter of the fistula is increased to 4 mm.

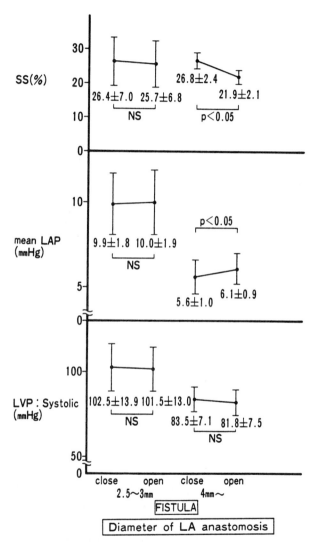

Fig. 5. When the size of the fistula is 2.5 to 3.0 mm, no significant changes in systolic shortening (SS%), mean left atrial pressure (LAP), and systolic left ventricular pressure (LVP) were observed. With the shunt 4 mm in diameter, a significant elevation of LAP and a drop in SS% are noted.

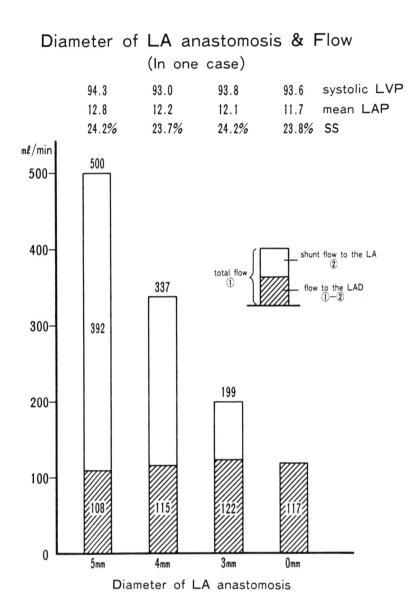

Fig. 6. Total graft flow volume and flow to the LAD with changes in the diameter of the fistula. Note the stable percentages in SS, LAP, and LVP measurements.

Conclusion

This alternative method may be useful to improve the patency of vein grafts to small or diffusely diseased coronary arteries. Still, caution using this method must be exercised. Other alternatives such as sequential grafting using the internal mammary artery (IMA) or gastroepiploic artery need to be considered first since they may provide better long-term benefit for the patient than any method using venous conduits.

References

1. Grondin CM, Limet R. Sequential anastomoses in coronary artery grafting: technical aspects and early and late angiographic results. Ann Thorac Surg 1977; 23:1–8.
2. Sewell WH, Sewell KV. Technique for the coronary snake graft operation. Ann Thorac Surg 1976; 22:58–65.
3. Dardik H, Sussman B, Ibrahim IM, Kahn M, et al. Distal arteriovenous fistula as an adjunct to maintaining arterial and graft patency for limb salvage. Surgery 1983; 94:478–486.
4. Blaisdell FW, Lim RC Jr, Hall AD, Thomas AN. Revascularization of severely ischemic extremities with an arteriovenous fistula. Am J Cardiol 1966; 121:166–171.
5. Spampinato N, Stassano P. Surgical A-V fistula in aortocoronary snake graft: preliminary report. J Cardiovasc Surg 1988; 29:100–102.

Part VI
Nonconduit Revascularization Techniques

Chapter 23

Patching Techniques for Coronary Artery Revascularization

Ronald K. Grooters and Hiroshi Nishida

The Coronary Ostial Patch

In 1965, Effler and colleagues[1] first reported a technique of patch angioplasty of the left main coronary artery (LMCA). Four out of nine patients (44%) died of the procedure. In 1970, these same coworkers[2] reported using a pericardial patch-graft technique for an LMCA stenosis but discontinued the procedure because of a 65% mortality rate. Hitchcock et al.[3] revived the patch angioplasty in 1983, with excellent results. Improved myocardial preservation and perioperative management, not available to Effler and colleagues, along with adherence to strict clinical and operative criteria made success possible using this technique. Other authors have subsequently described successful case reports (Table 1). Dion et al.[4,5] suggest that 1% of patients could be considered for this technique for either the left or right coronary ostia.

Pathology

Isolated coronary ostial stenosis is uncommon.[6] Found in less than 1% of patients, it seems to be seen more frequently in females.[7] The right coronary ostium may be more commonly affected,[8] probably because it is subjected to higher physiological stress when com-

From Grooters RK and Nishida H: (editors): *Alternative Bypass Conduits and Methods for Surgical Coronary Revascularization.* © Futura Publishing Co., Inc., Armonk, NY, 1994.

Table 1
Current Reports of Surgical Angioplasty

Author (Date)	Etiology of Stenosis	Ostia & No. of Patches	Patch Material	Success Rate
Hitchcock[3] (1983)	atherosclerosis	LM* 9	vein	100%
De Carvalbo[20] (1984)	atherosclerosis	LM 1	vein	100%
Gallotti[21] (1985)	valve surgery	LM 1	vein	100%
Morgan[22] (1987)	Takayasu's disease	LM,RCA** 2	pericardium	100%
Deuvaert[23] (1988)	atherosclerosis	LM 2	vein	100%
Villemot[17] (1988)	atherosclerosis	LM++ 35	vein—28 pericardium—7	100%
Dion[4] (1990)	atherosclerosis	LM 13	vein	} 78.3%+
		LM 9	pericardium }	
De Salazar[24] (1990)	atherosclerosis	LM 1	vein	100%
Eng[25] (1991)	atherosclerosis	LM 1	vein	} 100%
		RCA 2	vein }	
Nakano[18] (1992)	Takayasu's	LM 1	pericardium	100%

*LM—left main coronary artery; **RCA—right coronary artery; + failures, including death from air embolism; ++ endarterectomy performed with all angioplasties

pared to the left coronary artery ostium. Before the 1960s, syphilitic aortitis[9] was a common cause of ostial stenosis. Now atherosclerosis is the most frequently diagnosed etiology of LMCA stenosis, with an incidence as high as 7%[10] in patients with advanced coronary atherosclerosis. Other causes of ostial stenosis, although rare, include a congenital membrane,[11] fusion of the aortic leaflet to the aortic wall,[12] and Takayasu's aortitis.[13] Direct injury with subsequent stenosis following perfusion of a coronary artery during an aortic valve replacement or injection of cardioplegia using a balloon tip catheter[14] has also been reported. Such injuries have been reduced by improvements in the design of the catheters. More recently, left main stenosis has been reported following percutaneous transluminal coronary angioplasty (PTCA).[15,16] We have seen this complication in four patients over the past 2 years. In all of these cases, it has been diagnosed within the first 6 months following a PTCA and required coronary bypass surgery.

Detection

The diagnosis of an ostial stenosis is not always easy, but if it cannot be directly visualized by angiography, it should be suspected if there is difficulty cannulating the vessel or if there is a drop in distal coronary arterial pressure after insertion of the diagnostic cannula through the ostium. The absence of a reflux of contrast material into the sinus of Valsalva as the coronary artery is injected is another clue that an ostial lesion may be present.

Operative Technique and Results

Total cardiopulmonary bypass is used for all operations. The aorta is crossclamped, and the heart is arrested with a cold cardioplegia solution of the surgeon's preference. An aortotomy is made, similar to that for an aortic valve replacement. The incision then can be carried posteriorly onto the LMCA or anteriorly. The posterior approach (Fig. 1A) was used by Hitchcock et al. with success.[3] The aorta was retracted to the left, allowing easy access to the LMCA up to the bifurcation. The aortotomy was extended posteriorly into the orifice of the LMCA, across the stenosis, and into the origin of the left anterior descending (LAD) if necessary (Fig. 1B). The onlay patch of saphenous vein (SV) was then used to enlarge the diameter of the LMCA (Fig. 1C) and sutured with 6-0 Prolene. The patch is brought 2–3 cm onto the side of the aorta, and the rest of the aortotomy is closed with a running 3-0 or 4-0 Prolene.

The lumen measured between 3.5 and 4.5 mm after the technique. Endarterectomy was not done. Eight out of nine patients were free of angina at a follow-up, with a mean of 1.9 years. Calcification of the LMCA or additional lesions of the LAD and/or circumflex (CX) coronary arteries were considered contraindications to the patch procedure. All patients had normal ventricular function. The right coronary ostia patching could also be done by a similar technique (Fig. 2, A & B). For his last 12 patients, Dion et al.[4,5] preferred an anterior

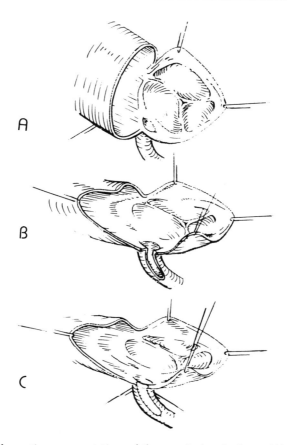

Fig. 1. Schematic representation of the surgical technique. (A) The aorta is opened into the left coronary sinus. (B) The incision is taken into the left coronary ostium, across the stenosis, and onto the origin of the left anterior descending (LAD) coronary artery. (C) A piece of saphenous vein (SV) is used as an onlay patch and brought onto the side of the aorta for a few millimeters to ensure a widely patent ostium (from Hitchcock JF et al.[3]).

approach to patch the LMCA (Fig. 2A). The right coronary ostium was patched simultaneously as necessary. The incision was started on the anterior aspect of the aorta and extended to the left lateral wall of the LMCA. The main pulmonary artery was retracted to the left and/or divided if need be. This allowed easy exposure of the anterior surface of the LMCA and its branches. The incision could then be made across the stenosis. The onlay patch could then be used to enlarge the ostium by bringing the patch onto the aorta (Fig. 2B).

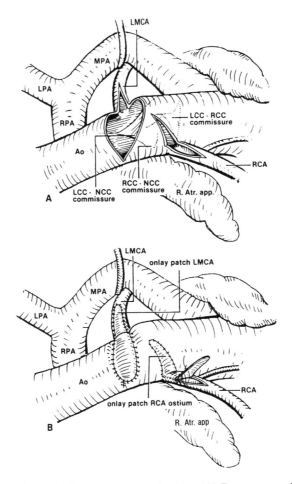

Fig. 2. Operative technique—a surgeon's view. (A) Exposure and incision of the left main coronary artery (LCMA) and of the right coronary artery (RCA) ostium. (B) After suture of onlay patches. MPA: main pulmonary artery; LPA: left pulmonary artery; RPA: right pulmonary artery; Ao: aorta; R. atr. App.: right atrial appendage; LCC-RCC commissure: commissure between the left coronary and right coronary aortic cusps; RCC-NCC commissure: commissure between the right coronary and noncoronary aortic cusps; LCC-NCC commissure: commissure between the left coronary and noncoronary aortic cusps (from Dion R, et al.[5]).

Transpulmonary Artery Approach

Villemot and colleagues[17] have successfully used a technique involving transection of the main coronary artery and its branches. Endarterectomy was also performed for all left main stenoses; in 28 patients a venous patch angioplasty was performed and in seven patients, the pericardium was used for the angioplasty. The latter material is now preferred.

Technique

The pulmonary artery trunk (PAT) is dissected from the aorta and transsected above the pulmonary cusps (Fig. 3). The proximal and distal ends of the PAT are easily retracted to expose the LMCA from its origin to the CX and LAD branches. An aortotomy is made 1 cm above the LMCA orifice and extended through the LMCA and its stenosis onto one of the branches, if necessary. The endarterectomy is either total or partial, depending on the extent of the disease, and may be continued onto the proximal branches of the LAD or CX. A pericardial or a venous patch is then sutured to enlarge the lumen of the LMCA to more than 4 mm and its branches to more than 3 mm. To test for leaks of the angioplasty, a crystalloid cardioplegia solution is injected under pressure into the ascending aorta before continuity of the PAT is restored.

The SV was used in the first 14 patients, but fresh autologous pericardial patch is now preferred and has been used in the last nine patients. Thromboendarterectomy, at times, is unavoidable (it was used in five patients), but with the anterior approach it seems much easier and safer. Dion et al.,[4] as well as Nakano and associates,[18] have used this approach in combination with aortic valve replacement. One of Nakano's patients had Takayasu's disease of the LMCA. This technique was felt to be better than an aortocoronary bypass graft because the aortic wall was severely thickened to 4–5 mm from a fibrous reaction. Late occlusion of the proximal anastomosis secondary to intimal proliferation of the aortitis was felt to be a likely possibility if conventional aortocoronary bypass was used.

Theoretical Advantages

(1) With conventional coronary bypass grafting, there may be some loss of perfusion pressure retrograde to the anastomosis. This

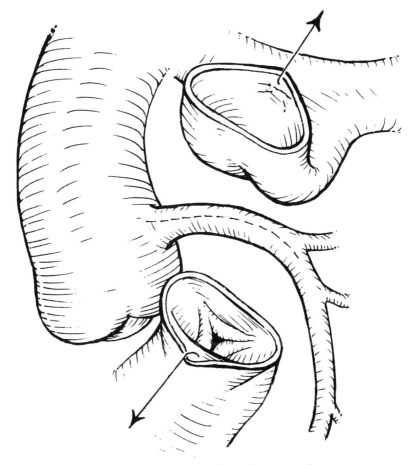

Fig. 3. The left main coronary artery (LMCA): the transpulmonary artery approach (from Villemot JP, et al[17]).

decrease of the pressure head is possible from a phenomenon known as the Prizometer principle (Fig. 4). Theoretically, a patch of the left main stenosis would restore the antegrade flow pattern and thus provide superior coronary perfusion.

(2) Flow from routine coronary artery grafting is not necessary for isolated osteal stenosis, and thus the osteal stenosis would not thrombose and produce a graft-dependent heart that is frequently seen with the usual venous or arterial coronary artery grafts.

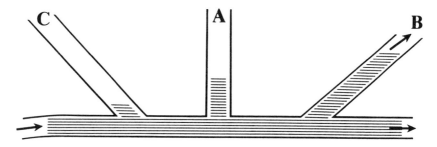

Fig. 4. Prizometer principle. Limb C of this experimental model shows a much lower pressure head with retrograde perfusion compared with limb B, which is being perfused antegradely.

(3) Native coronary ostia are somewhat protected from the aortic systolic pressure wave. By contrast, an aortocoronary saphenous vein graft (SVG) would be subject to the arterial pressure wave, which may predispose the SVG to accelerated graft atherosclerosis.

(4) Conventional bypass grafting uses a significant amount of graft conduit (venous or arterial), whereas the angioplasty uses very little or none, if the pericardium is preferred.

(5) Direct surgical patch angioplasty could allow for a PTCA if distal coronary stenosis later developed. It would also be much easier to pass a catheter through the wide-open patched ostia than to try a PTCA through a vein graft, which is frequently diseased.

Clinical Guidelines for Patch Angioplasty

(1) Isolated proximal lesions of the left main and right coronary ostia are ideal. Surgeons report that they proceed cautiously if the lesions involve a long segment of the LMCA or are some distance from the ostia. Dion et al.[4,5] have extended the patch angioplasty to the middle and/or distal stenoses of the LMCA with a 90% success rate in ten patients. They prefer the anterior approach (Fig. 2) for better exposure.

(2) Calcification on the coronary angiogram is a contraindication to the procedure. However, the absence of visible calcification does not preclude having to deal with the calcification intraoperatively and may force the use of endarterectomy. Dion et al.[4] reported that 34.8% of patients with no angiographic calcification still had significant calcification that required a localized thromboendarterectomy. Most of these procedures were successful, even with calcium present.

(3) Good ventricular function was initially felt to be a must.[3] With better techniques, such as retrograde cardioplegia, poor left-ventricular function should be less of a problem. Dion et al.[4] have applied this procedure to patients with less than desirable ventricular function and feel that it is only a relative contraindication.

(4) Most authors used age (limited to those less than 60 years old) as a criterion when considering the patch angioplasty. Dion et al.[4] has reported attempting seven angioplasties in six patients greater than 60 years of age, with only three of seven angioplasties succeeding. The patch angioplasty can be considered in patients older than 60 if no calcification is identified on the preoperative angiogram and if conventional grafting is likely to be unsatisfactory.

(5) The need for endarterectomy is likely, and it can be used successfully for the extensively diseased LMCA. Dion et al.[4] have used endarterectomy when they have had to, but Mujamoto,[19] unlike many other surgeons[20-24] aggressively used this approach for extensively diseased LMCAs in conjunction with bypass grafts to distal branches. He felt that this lowered the incidence of incomplete revascularization of the left coronary system to 5%.

Unique Complications

(1) The possibility of air embolization in the postoperative period was reported by Dion et al.[4] This is an increased possibility because of the open aorta, and air could become trapped in the ventricle. Care must be taken to vent for air as much as possible.

(2) When performing an anterior LMCA angioplasty, one must be careful to avoid kinking of the onlay patch at the site where the LMCA and the left posterolateral aortic wall meet.[4] Narrowing or occlusion of the new ostium could result, particularly with the anterior approach.

(3) When attempting this technique, the surgeon must be very careful not to leave any intimal flap. This occurs most frequently when the surgeon is forced to use thromboendarterectomy. A flap could lead to a disastrous thrombosis at the ostia.

Conclusion

The limits of the coronary ostia angioplasty and the conditions for its use are nearly established. Clinical situations, such as the absence of conduits or the failure to find a major branch of the LMCA to bypass may necessitate that the surgeon use this part of his armamentarium. It may well be that this technique would be useful in about 1% of patients requiring coronary revascularization.

The Ascending Aortic Patch

Technical problems created by the extreme differences of wall thickness between the new coronary graft (vein or artery) and the ascending aorta have been implicated as a cause of early graft failure. The ascending aortic wall patch can be a simple and safe method to assist the surgeon in the construction of the proximal aortic anastomosis. Alternative methods such as suturing the graft to the hood of a proximal SVG,[25] constructing a composite graft to an in situ internal mammary artery (IMA) graft,[26,27] and placing the proximal end of the graft elsewhere, such as the innominate artery[28] or another proximal coronary artery[29] are other satisfactory methods, but the patch technique of the ascending aorta may occasionally be a useful alternative as part of the surgeon's repertoire.

The Patch and the Free IMA Technique

The proximal anastomoses between the aorta and the free IMA is constructed after completion of all distal anastomoses. The cross-clamp is then released and the heart is perfused and rewarmed while on cardiopulmonary bypass. After the partial occlusion, the clamp is applied to the ascending aorta and an oval piece of aorta (10 mm in diameter) is excised as described by Kanter et al.[30] (Fig. 5).

A generous piece of autologous pericardium or SV (if large enough) as described by Schimert[31] is sutured to the aortic defect using continuous 6-0 polypropylene suture. A 4 mm aortic punch is then used to create a circular opening in the center of the patch. The proximal end of the free IMA graft is then spatulated and anastomosed to the pericardial patch using continuous 7-0 polypropylene suture.

Technical Modification for the Thickened Aorta

If the ascending aorta has a large calcified or severely thickened atherosclerotic plaque on its anterior surface, proximal anastomosis of the SVG may be technically difficult to perform. Robiscek[32] has

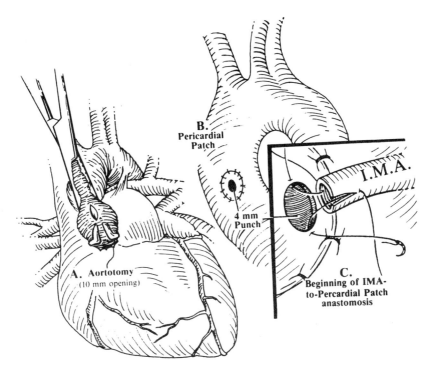

Fig. 5. Technique of proximal anastomosis with pericardium for free internal mammary artery (IMA) grafts. (A) A partial occlusion clamp is applied, and a 10 mm oval of aorta is excised. (B) A generous patch of autologous pericardium is sewn to the defect with continuous 6-0 polypropylene suture. A 4 mm defect is created in the pericardial patch using an aortic punch. (C) The proximal free IMA graft is spatulated and anastomosed to the pericardial patch using continuous 7-0 polypropylene sutures (from Kanter KR, et al.[30]).

successfully sutured a large oval patch of Teflon cloth to a diseased ascending aorta to which the vein grafts were anastomosed. The oval patch was made approximately 3 cm. in length and 1.5 cm. in width to which the proximal SVG anastomoses were sutured using 6-0 polypropylene suture. The appropriate number of holes measuring 2.5 mm in diameter were burned in the center line of the fabric with a glowing iron. The ascending aorta was side clamped with a partial occluding clamp, and a longitudinal incision the length of the patch was made on the anterior surface of the aorta. The patch carrying the SVG was sutured onto the longitudinal slit with 4-0 polypropylene suture reinforced with a narrow strip of Teflon felt (Fig. 6).

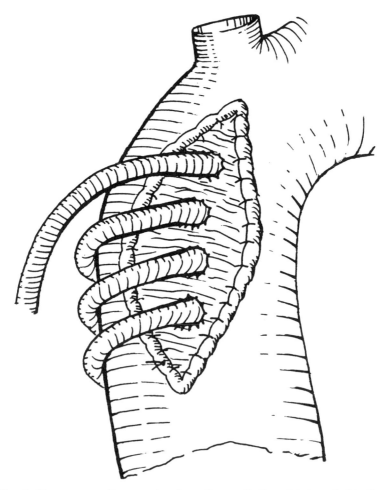

Fig. 6. Coronary grafts emerging from the synthetic patch inserted in the ascending aorta (from Robiscek F, et al.[32]).

This technique was successful in two patients, one with three proximal anastomoses and another with four proximal anastomoses. Robiscek et al.[32] commented that vein-aortic graft anastomoses have also worked for total aortic root replacements in which the coronary arteries required simultaneous grafting.

The "No Touch" Alternative

Not all ascending aortas with atherosclerotic plaque are amenable to a patch technique, and caution must be used in this decision. Some of the ascending aortas are completely calcified or atherosclerotic, making side clamping very hazardous. This atherosclerosis may extend into the lumen of the ascending aorta and may be very friable. This material, if disrupted, would then embolize to the brain or heart. The incidence of this type of aorta is not definitely known, but Peigh et al.[33] reported that only 6 out of 2,658 (0.2%) patients undergoing coronary artery bypass grafting had ascending aortic disease not amenable to receiving a proximal anastomosis. Mills et al.[34] has reported ascending aortic disease requiring a "no touch" technique in 16 out of 1,735 patients (0.9%).

Suma[35] was the first to report a "no touch" technique used on three patients. The technique utilized only in situ grafts of the IMAs and the right gastroepiploic artery (RGEA), fibrillatory arrest without an aortic crossclamp, and a left ventricular vent with femoral artery perfusion (Fig. 7). Peigh et al.[33] constructed the proximal anastomoses of vein grafts onto the proximal IMAs end-to-side (Chapter 15, Fig. 1). We have also used this technique of composite grafts in four patients successfully without evidence of perioperative stroke. It is very important to maintain a high index of suspension for the severely diseased aorta so that the "no touch" technique can be considered before the ascending aorta is violated with a crossclamp or side clamp. Echocardiography of the ascending aorta as well as aortography may be useful to confirm this severe condition so an alternative "no touch" method can be planned.[36]

The Trap of the Crossclamped Diseased Ascending Aorta

Nearly every surgeon has applied the crossclamp to the ascending aorta only to find by palpation an extremely thickened irregular

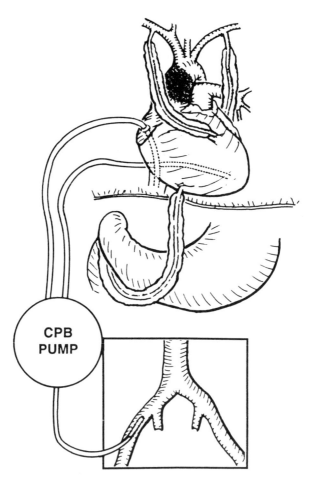

Fig. 7. Scheme of the aortic no-touch technique: maximal utilization of in situ arterial grafts using bilateral internal mammary and gastroepiploic arteries, fibrillatory arrest without an aortic clamp, left ventricular vent, and femoral artery perfusion. (CPB = cardiopulmonary bypass) (from Suma H[35]).

diseased structure (Fig. 8A). This problem, most of the time, can be handled by performing the proximal anastomosis with the cross-clamp left on the ascending aorta but only if (1) no atherosclerotic debris is detected coming from the aortic incision and (2) a supple area in the aorta is found. If the surgeon suddenly finds copious amounts of atherosclerotic debris floating from the aortotomy (Fig. 8B), the chance of a cerebrovascular event from this condition is almost certain. To avoid a perioperative stroke in this situation, we have opened the aorta in a "soft" area wide enough to debride all potentially friable plaque (Fig. 8C). Once the entire ascending aorta proximal to the crossclamp is debrided and washed vigorously, horizontal pledgeted mattress sutures of 3-0 polypropylene are placed in the aortotomy (Fig. 8D). Proximal anastomoses are performed on a supple nondiseased portion of the aorta, adjacent to the aortotomy, if possible. The crossclamp is then released with the aorta remaining open for two or three seconds while the cardiopulmonary bypass pump is still at a flow rate of 3–4 liters/min (Fig. 8E). This flushes through the aortotomy any debris caught within the crossclamp. The pump is then stopped, and the mattress sutures are quickly tied (Fig. 8F). The pump is then restarted, and the original flow rate is maintained during rewarming. *No further clamping of the aorta is done.* We have encountered three such situations, and by using this technique none of the patients developed evidence of perioperative stroke.

Conclusion

The ascending aorta, particularly if diseased, will continue to be a challenge for the surgeon. The ascending aortic patch may be helpful, but this is not the only answer. "No touch" techniques of the aorta are very useful, particularly if combined with the alternative bypass techniques of placing the vein or arterial graft proximal anastomosis onto other arterial structures—such as the in situ proximal IMA, the innominate artery, or a normal coronary artery—or by using all in situ arterial grafts.

The Coronary Artery Saphenous Vein Patch-IMA Bypass

The SV bypass graft has been used successfully as a vein graft patch to revascularize a long, endarterectomized coronary artery.[37]

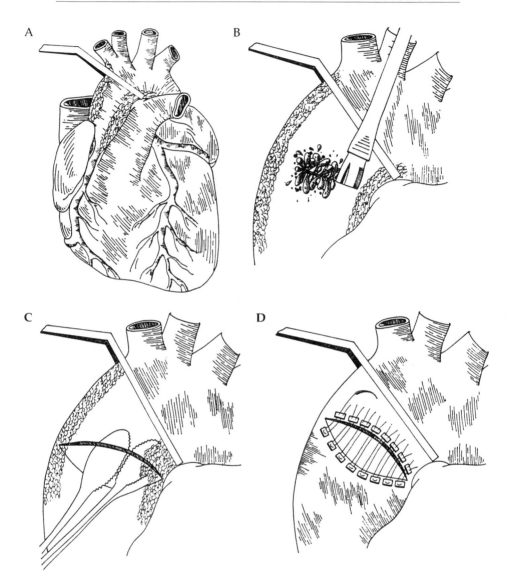

Fig. 8. A method of coping with the trap of the crossclamped diseased ascending aorta. (A) Crossclamping of the ascending aorta with undetected friable atherosclerosis. (B) Detecting friable debris but not until the aorta has been opened. (C) Extending the incision to inspect and remove friable debris. (D) Placing horizontal sutures to close the large incision. (Continued)

E

F

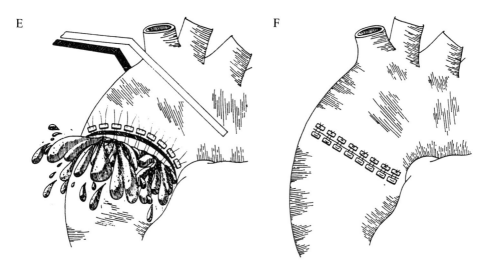

Fig. 8, continued. (E) Release of the crossclamp to flush debris, possibly caught in the crossclamp, through the large incision. (F) Cardiopulmonary bypass is shut down during a brief period to tie the sutures or at least pull them together. No more clamps are applied.

The SVG with its lower patency rate when compared to an IMA graft is then accepted. A unique technique described by Ladowski and associates[38] has successfully used the SV patch to a long endarterectomy of the LAD but then has revascularized this combination with an IMA. This tailored SV patch avoids a patulous lumen and flow discrepancies and also expedites the distal IMA anastomosis. In addition, the thrombogenicity of a coronary artery with the entire lumen having undergone an endarterectomy is eliminated. The main benefit may be the contribution of the long-term benefit of the IMA to this difficult situation, but further follow-up is needed. The short-term results are excellent, with 17 out of 18 patients free of angina at an average follow-up time of 12 months. Two patients suffered postoperative myocardial infarctions.

Technique

Ladowski et al.[38] suggested that this technique be used when the LAD is completely calcified, and a suitable area for construction of an anastomosis with an IMA cannot be found. The LAD is opened

1–2 cm, and an endarterectomy is performed. If a 1.5 mm probe does not pass freely or if an endarterectomy margin is unacceptable, a more extensive endarterectomy is performed (Fig. 9, a–c). The diagonal arteries are frequently included in the arteriotomy. Direct visualization of the entire endarterectomy is preferred, rather than resorting to a traction endarterectomy of the atheromatous plaque.

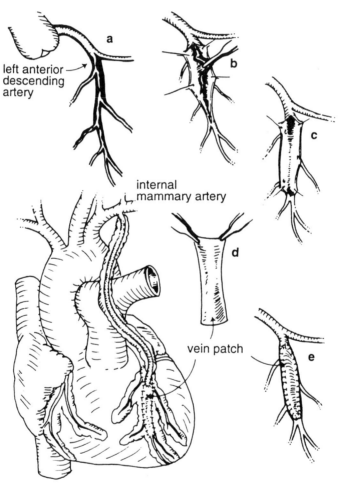

Fig. 9. Endarterectomy, reconstruction, and bypass of the anterior descending coronary artery (from Ladowski JS, et al.[38]).

A vein graft patch is then tailored to accommodate the arteriotomy and sutured in place with 6-0 or 7-0 continuous polypropylene suture. The width of the patch is trimmed to avoid a patulous LAD-vein patch lumen. The desired reconstructed LAD is depicted in Figure 9e. Cardioplegia is again administered at this time to provide myocardial protection and to assess hemostasis. The IMA is then anastomosed to a 3–5 mm longitudinal incision in the vein patch, using continuous 8-0 polypropylene to complete the graft (Fig. 9). An important point to be made is that patency of the proximal part of the bypassed artery is not desirable. Competitive flow with the IMA graft is to be avoided; therefore, proximal disease in the artery bypass is not removed.

Postoperative care included anticoagulation with Heparin in the immediate postoperative period and continued with Coumadin (warfarin sodium), maintaining a prothrombin time of 1.25 to 1.5 times control for 3 months. Aspirin is continued after Coumadin is discontinued.

Other options for reconstruction of a long arteriotomy exist. Complete proximal endarterectomy with a simple closure or vein patch closure is an option usually avoided. The creation of a long SV to LAD anastomosis using the vein graft as the bypass conduit is probably the most common technique, but then the benefits of the IMA are not present, and vein graft stenosis can be the result (Chapter 24, Fig. 3). A limited arteriotomy with a traction endarterectomy, followed by a graft of the arteriotomy, is another useful option. This conceivably produces a coronary artery lumen totally without intima that may be more thrombogenic. Another option, which can be very difficult and time consuming, is the lengthy anastomosis of the IMA to the lengthy coronary artery endarterectomy. All these options are viable, but this IMA-vein patch technique described by Ladowski et al.[38] seems very logical for the difficult, diffusely diseased coronary artery.

References

1. Effler DB, Sones FM, Favaloro R, Groves LK. Coronary endarterectomy with patch graft reconstruction: clinical experience with 34 cases. Ann Surg 1965; 162:590–601.
2. Favaloro RG, Effler DB, Groves LK, Sheldon WC, et al. Severe segmental obstruction of the left main coronary and its division. surgical treatment by the saphenous vein graft technique. J Thorac Cardiovasc Surg 1970; 60:469–482.

3. Hitchcock JF, Robles de Medina EO, Jambroes G. Angioplasty of the left main coronary artery for isolated left main coronary artery disease. J Thorac Cardiovasc Surg 1983; 85:880–884.

4. Dion R, Verhelst R, Matta A, Rosseau M, et al. Surgical angioplasty of the left main coronary artery. J Thorac Cardiovasc Surg 1990; 99:241–250.

5. Dion R, Puts JP. Bilateral surgical ostial angioplasty of the right and left coronary arteries. J Thorac Cardiovasc Surg 1991; 102;643–645.

6. Hutter JA, Pasaogbe I, Williams BT. The incidence and management of coronary ostial stenosis. J Cardiovasc Surg 1985; 26:581–584.

7. Thompson R. Isolated coronary ostial stenosis in women. J Am Coll Cardiol 1986; 7:997–1003.

8. Enos WF, Beyer JC, Holmes RH. Arteriosclerosis of the aortic sinuses. Am J Clin Pathol 1963; 39:506–511.

9. Scharman WB, Wallach JB, Anguist A. Myocardial infarctions due to syphilitic coronary ostial stenosis. Am Heart J 1950; 40:603–613.

10. DeMots H, Rosch J, McAnulty JH, Rahimtoola SH. Left main coronary artery disease. Cardiovasc Clin 1977; 8:201–211.

11. Josa M, Danielson GK, Weidman WH, Edwards WD. Congenital ostial membrane of left main coronary artery. J Thorac Cardiovasc Surg 1981; 81:338–346.

12. Waxman MB, Kong Y, Behar VS, Sabiston DC, et al. Fusion of left aortic cusp to the aortic wall with occlusion of the left coronary ostium and aortic stenosis and insufficiency. Circulation 1970; 41:849–857.

13. Chun PKC, Jones R, Robinowitz M, Davia JE, et al. Coronary ostial stenosis in Takayasu's arteritis. Chest 1980; 78:330–331.

14. Midell AI, Deboer A, Bermudja G. Postperfusion coronary ostial stenosis: incidence and significance. J Thorac Cardiovasc Surg 1976; 72:80–85.

15. Graf RH, Verani MS. Left main coronary artery stenosis: a possible complication of transluminal coronary angioplasty. Cathet Cardiovasc Diagn 1984; 10:163–166.

16. Wayne VS, Harper RW, Pitt A. Left main coronary artery stenosis after percutaneous transluminal coronary angioplasty. Am J Cardiol 1988; 61:459–460.

17. Villemot JP, Godiner JPL, Peiffert B, Zamorano J, et al. Endarterectomy of the left main coronary artery stenosis by a "transpulmonary artery approach." Eur J CardioThorac Surg 1988; 2:453–457.

18. Nakano S, Yasuhisa S, Mitounoi K, Taniquchi K, et al. Transaortic patch angioplasty for left coronary ostial stenosis in a patient with Takayasu's aortitis. Ann Thorac Surg 1992; 53:694–695.

19. Mujamoto AT. Discussion of Dion et al.[4] J Thorac Cardiovasc Surg 1990; 99:249–250.

20. De Carvalbo RG, Ribeiro EJ, Brofman PR, Da Rocha Loure DR. Angioplastia cirurgiaa do ostio da arterea coronaria esquerda relato de caso. Arq Bras Cardiol 1984; 42(5):355–360.

21. Gallotti R, Ornaghi D, Panisi P, Verna E, et al. Angioplastica del tronco comsine della coronorea sinistra con patch venoso. G Ital Cardiol 1985; 15(I):414–416.

22. Morgan JM, Honey M, Pray HH, Belcher P, et al. Angina pectoris in a case of Takayasu's disease: revascularization by coronary ostioplasty and bypass grafting. Eur Heart J 1987; 8:1354–1358.

23. Deuvaert FE, De Paepe J, Van Nooten G, Peperstraeste B, et al. Transaortic saphenous vein patch angioplasty for left main coronary artery stenosis. J Cardiovasc Surg 1988; 29:610–613

24. De Salazar AO, Aromendi JI, Juanena C, Onate A, et al. Angioplastia un parche en estenosis aislada del tronco de la arteria coronaria izquierda. Rev Esp Cardiol 1990; 43:417–419.

25. Eng J, Beton DC, Lawson RAM, Moussalli H, et al. Coronary ostial stenosis: surgical considerations. Int J Cardiol 1991; 30:285–288.

26. Bainer HB. The internal mammary artery as a free graft. J Thorac Cardiovasc Surg 1973; 66:219.

27. Mills N. Physiologic and technical aspects of internal mammary artery–coronary artery bypass grafts. In: Cohn LH, ed. Modern Technics in Surgery: Cardiac/Thoracic Surgery. Mt. Kisco, NY: Futura Publishing Co. Inc., 1982: 48–17.

28. Weinstein G, Killen DA. Innominate artery-coronary artery bypass graft in a patient with calcific aortitis. J Thorac Cardiovasc Surg 1980; 79:312–313.

29. Nishida H, Soltanzadeh H, Grooters RK, Thieman KC. Coronary-coronary bypass using internal mammary artery. Ann Thorac Surg 1988; 46:577–578.

30. Kanter KR, Barner HB. Improved technique for the proximal anastomosis with free internal mammary artery grafts. Ann Thorac Surg 1987; 44:556–557.

31. Schimert G, Vidne BA, Lee AB Jr. Free internal mammary artery graft: an improved surgical technique. Ann Thorac Surg 1975; 19:474–477.

32. Robiscek F, Rubenstein RB. Calcification and thickening of the aortic wall complicating aortocoronary grafting: a technical modification. Ann Thorac Surg 1980; 29:84–85.

33. Peigh PS, Di Sesa VJ, Collins JJ Jr, Cohn LH. Coronary bypass grafting with totally calcified or acutely dissected ascending aorta. Ann Thorac Surg 1991; 51:102–104.

34. Mills NL, Everson CT. Atherosclerosis of the ascending aorta and coronary artery bypass: pathology, clinical correlates, and operative management. J Thorac Cardiovasc Surg 1991; 102:546–553.

35. Suma H. Coronary artery bypass grafting in patients with calcified ascending aorta: aorta no touch technique. Ann Thorac Surg 1989; 728–730.

36. Marshall WG, Barzelai B, Kouchoukos NT, Soffity J. Intraoperative ultrasonic imaging of the ascending aorta. Ann Thorac Surg 1989; 48:339–344.

37. Brenowitz JB, Kayser KL, Johnson WD. Results of coronary endarterectomy and reconstruction. J Thorac Cardiovasc Surg 1988; 95:1–10.

38. Ladowski JS, Schalylien MH, Underhill DJ, Peterson AC. Endarterectomy, vein patch, and mammary bypass of the anterior descending artery. Ann Thorac Surg 1991; 52:1187–1189.

Chapter 24

Extensive Coronary Artery Endarterectomy

Pablo Pedraza

The first successful coronary endarterectomy was performed by Bailey and associates[1] in 1956 without cardiopulmonary bypass by using a method of retrograde curettage made possible by an instrument developed by May.[2] Soon after, Longmire and colleagues[3] in 1958 and Sabiston and Blalock[4] in 1961 reported success with a direct approach by incising directly over the plaque and then manually removing it. By 1964, Effler and colleagues[5] reported using cardiopulmonary bypass with profound hypothermia to perform the endarterectomy and then repair the arteriotomy with a vein patch. By 1967, their series had grown to 71 patients with a successful surgical outcome for 60 patients.[6] Ever since these initial studies, other surgeons have subsequently reported on their extensive experiences,[7–9] concluding that this controversial and challenging procedure is an appropriate adjunct to bypass grafting in selected patients (Table 1).

The primary indication for coronary endarterectomy is the presence of diffuse, obstructive coronary atherosclerosis. This brings up the issue of the exact definition of diffuse coronary disease, which still has not been well defined. However, those vessels containing multiple areas of an irregularly narrowed "rosarylike" angiographic appearance, significantly obstructing the artery (greater than 70% of the lumen), potentially qualify as vessels for the possible consideration of endarterectomy. Also, at the time of surgery, it may be determined that endarterectomy is necessary because the degree of

From Grooters RK and Nishida H: (editors): *Alternative Bypass Conduits and Methods for Surgical Coronary Revascularization.* © Futura Publishing Co., Inc., Armonk, NY, 1994.

251

Table 1
Results of Endarterectomy—Three Largest Series

Author (date reported)	No. of patients	Operative mortality (percent)	Perioperative MI	Patency rate (no. of grafts)	Clinical improvement— percent asymptomatic	Percent Late survival
Livesay[8] (1986)	3,369	4.4% 6.4% (1970–1976) 3.5% (1977–1984)	5.4%	—	52% at 5 yrs 32% at 10 yrs	86% at 5 yrs 67% at 10 yrs
Brenowitz[10] (1988)	1,255*	6.3*	6.5%*	early+ 88.9% (801/901)	*65.5% at 51.4 mos	*92% at 5 yrs
	1,246**	10.4%**	13.1%**	late++ 71.1% (137/191)	**66.3% at 43.9 mos	**83.8% at 5 yrs
Keon[9] (1988)	1,718	6.5%	10.0%	1 yr 73% 5 yrs 62% 10 yrs 51%	81% at 5 yrs 72% at 8 yrs	73% at 12 yrs

*—one endarterectomy per patient; **—multiple endarterectomies per patient; +—early; ++—late—average of 31.4 mos

atherosclerosis is such that a standard bypass graft may be compromised by local disease at the planned graft site on the coronary artery. Additionally, coronary artery runoff may be considered in jeopardy if diffuse "downstream" atherosclerosis is suspected by palpation and by probing. With these findings, alternatives such as splitting the plaque with patch grafting or multiple sequential grafting techniques must also be considered. In spite of the increased surgical risk,[8,10] coronary endarterectomy seems to demonstrate beneficial long-term effects as well as salvage patients previously considered inoperable. As surgeons are seeing more patients with diffuse peripheral coronary artery disease, effective revascularization will be increasingly impossible without the resurgence of coronary artery endarterectomy as an alternative in a surgeon's armamentarium.

Technique

Coronary endarterectomy requires a significant degree of discipline and commitment since once the decision has been made to increase blood supply to the coronary artery bed by this technique, turning back is not an option. Optimal surgical technique, extracorporeal perfusion, and myocardial protection may vary for each surgeon and are essential inseparable interwoven elements of successful coronary revascularization, particularly when endarterectomy is included. The main principle that each surgeon needs to follow with this procedure is that the complete removal of the atherosclerotic plaque is imperative, even though it may be tedious and time consuming (Fig. 1).

Throughout the years, my approach has called for total cardiopulmonary bypass with double venous cannulation in the majority of cases with the additional use of an aortic vent. High flow in the range of 2.5 L/m^2/min along with high perfusion pressures in the range of 80–100 mm Hg are most favorable. Systemic hypothermia of only 34°C is used. Intermittent ischemic arrest by means of aortic crossclamping with a carefully followed average clamp time of 20 minutes is used. I have the perfusionists inform me of the time at 5 minute increments to estimate the necessary sequence of events during the endarterectomy procedure. Rarely, the time is extended to 25 minutes. Once this ischemic time is used, the crossclamp is released, and the heart is perfused for a minimum of 5 minutes. This time period is carefully followed, but occasionally extra minutes are given to assure

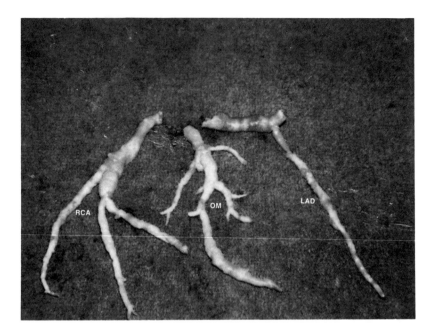

Fig. 1. Removal of diffuse atherosclerotic plaque of all three vessels. RCA: right coronary artery; OM: obtuse marginal; LAD: left anterior descending. Note that the branch to the first diagonal is not present but was also endarterectomized.

optimal recovery of the myocardium. In general, the heart is kept beating when the crossclamp is off, but when the clamp is reapplied, cardiac arrest by means of electrical fibrillation with DC current may be necessary to assure a quiet operative field. Since 1983, nifedipine in varying dosages has been used systemically in all patients, and the use of allopurinol, usually 300 mg the evening before surgery, has also become routine.

I am comfortable with the intermittent aortic clamping technique, also used by other surgeons in the Milwaukee, Wisconsin, area. This is also known as ischemic arrest and is used to obtain a bloodless and motionless surgical field of cardiac asystole. Other methods of myocardial preservation may also be appropriate, such as the use of cold blood cardioplegia, which provides good myocardial protection.[11,12] However, my personal experience in this regard is quite limited, and when crystalloid cardioplegia has been used, I have had difficulty distinguishing tissue planes of the endarterectomy. Retrograde coronary sinus perfusion has also been successfully reported for extensive coronary endarterectomy[13] and may be a more convenient method of myocardial protection since it can be continuous or instituted anytime during a sometimes prolonged procedure.

Upon examination of the heart for the potential use and extent of the endarterectomy, correlation of angiographic findings with visual inspection and careful palpation often yield information critical to the technical maneuvers necessary. These vessels are frequently calcified, and the extent of induration may offer guidance on the potential extent of the arteriotomy needed, as well as the length of specimen to be extracted. At the point of the most extensive atheromatous plaque, the epicardium is incised, and the longitudinal arteriotomy into the plaque is made. The plane of dissection between the outer media and the atherosclerotic plug is usually obvious. This plane is also identifiable by using blunt dissection with a small mosquito clamp or one of the jaws of the instrument. On occasion, the tip of a small, fine vascular forceps can also be used (Fig. 2). The dissection is continued proximally and distally to the endarterectomy incision. After dissecting and freeing the core proximally, it is divided, and the distal dissection is continued slowly and carefully. For the right coronary artery (RCA), mechanical extraction of the core, using rhythmic coordinating maneuvers of traction on the core and countertraction on the adventitia of the coronary artery or tissues surrounding the vessels is both necessary and safe.

The atheroma occasionally may be challenging since frequently it is heavily calcified, may be brittle, and will fracture easily. Rarely, some segments contain necrotic, soft "toothpastelike" debris. This requires careful attention, including irrigation, to prevent embolization. Retained debris, fronds, and loose material, when seen and identified, must be meticulously removed. Occasionally, a "milking" of the coronary branches is helpful to extract these potential emboli through the arteriotomy. Most often, the atheromatous material is extracted as one unit through a relatively small arteriotomy. Palpation of the distal vessels and its branches is recommended to insure that other areas of plaque have not been left behind. Endarterectomy of the left anterior descending (LAD), with its numerous branches (diagonals and septal perforators) coming from the LAD at planes perpendicular to each other, almost always requires a lengthy incision to assure complete core removal without disrupting atheromatous ex-

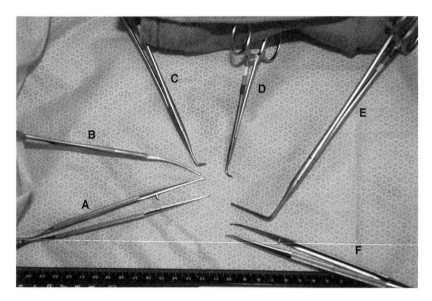

Fig. 2. Useful instruments for assisting with the endarterectomy. (A) micro endarterectomy forceps, 7¼ in, Scanlan, St. Paul, Minn. (B) plaque retriever, short—American V. Mueller, Chicago, Ill. (C) mini plaque retriever—American V. Mueller, Chicago, Ill. (D) Oschner forceps full curve 90° angle jaw, 4½ in, Scanlon, St. Paul, Minn. (E) plaque retriever, long—American V. Mueller, Chicago, Ill. (F) micro endarterectomy forceps, 7¼ in, curved—Scanlan, St. Paul, Minn.

tension into each branch. This is particularly necessary at the level of the first diagonal and first septal perforating branch.

An additional downstream arteriotomy is another consideration if the distal part of the plaque fractures, or it is technically necessary to provide an easier and complete endarterectomy. Marginal branches of the circumflex system are amendable to endarterectomy but sometimes have proven to be challenging experiences. I have, on rare occasions, performed an endarterectomy of the proximal circumflex through the left main coronary artery (LMCA) at bifurcation with the LAD. This dissection must be slow and meticulous. This can be done if the LMCA is long but should not be attempted if the vessel is short. In my experience, endarterectomy of the circumflex branch seems to be the most difficult and challenging of all, including its marginal branches. It is quite difficult to perform an endarterectomy safely in the atrioventricular groove, and it is usually not necessary.

The long arteriotomy is then closed with 7-0 polypropylene, usually as a distal anastomosis of the vein graft. This insures good inflow. Rarely is a vein patch used, although it has been reported[14] to be used successfully by providing inflow from an internal mammary artery (IMA) graft (Chapter 23). Another interesting technique used to assess and assure good distal runoff is the use of indocyanine green as reported by Keon and associates.[9] Twenty-five milligrams of dye is diluted in 200 mL of crystalloid cardioplegia solution of which 10–15 mL is injected through the vein grafts after the endarterectomy is complete. The distal vessels fill with green dye, and a green myocardial blush is seen in the perfused area, which technically indicates a successful endarterectomy.

Results

Operative Mortality

The operative mortality rates for patients receiving coronary artery endarterectomy vary widely, with a range of zero percent reported by Hockberg et al.[15] and Kuijpers et al.[16] for 25 and 32 patients, respectively, to 10% reported by Dumanian[17] and Wallash et al. [18] for 260 and 60 patients, respectively. The three latest studies with the largest numbers of patients (Table 1)[8–10] demonstrate 30-day perioperative mortality rates ranging from 4.4% to 10.4%.

Brenowitz and colleagues[10] stratified operative mortality rates according to risk factors (age over 70 years, repeat operation, insulin-dependent diabetes mellitus, female sex, and severe left ventricular function defined as ejection fraction 0.10 to 0.35) on one vs. multiple endarterectomies. If only one endarterectomy was done without other risk factors, the operative mortality rate was 1.7% vs. 5.3% if the patient had two or more risk factors. If multiple endarterectomies were performed, the mortality rates were 5.4% for patients with no risk factors, 9.9% for one risk factor present, and 26.9% for two or more risk factors present. Livesay and associates[8] also demonstrated an operative mortality rate of 8.5% for endarterectomy of the LAD versus 4.2% with endarterectomy of the other coronary arteries. This group of surgeons noted a substantial decrease of early mortality for patients done during the latter period of the study: 1970–1976 (6.4%) versus 1977–1984 (3.5%; $p < 0.01$). The operative mortality rate of Keon et al.,[9] although the highest of the three largest series at 6.5%, also included both elective and emergency coronary artery bypass procedures. In contrast, the operative mortality rates of Brenowitz et al.[10] and Livesay et al.[8] for coronary artery bypass without endarterectomy, including patients with risk factors, were significantly lower at 4.0% and 2.6%, respectively.

Perioperative Myocardial Infarction

The reported rates of perioperative myocardial infarction associated with coronary endarterectomy range from 5% to 30%.[8,19–21] The larger experiences (Table 1) have a narrower and lower range of 5.4% to 13%. The highest percentage (13%) is associated with multiple endarterectomies—three to seven per patient with an average of five. Different criteria used for the diagnosis of infarction may also account for the broad range of myocardial injuries, although most surgeons do report infarction rates for coronary artery bypass combined with endarterectomy to be at least twice that of coronary artery bypass alone.

Patency Rates

The two largest studies[9,10] (Table 1) have angiographically evaluated patency rates at different time periods after surgery. Brenowitz et al.[10] demonstrated in 940 patients an early graft patency of 801 out of 901 grafts (88.9%) for endarterectomy grafts, compared to 2,939 of 3,248 patent grafts (90.5%) conventional vein grafts. Late graft patency in 288 symptomatic patients (average 31.4 mo) was 137 out of 191 (71.1%) for endarterectomy grafts and 644 out of 850 (75.8%) for conventional vein grafts. The late graft patency for the RCA was 57 out of 82 (69.5%), for the LAD, 69 out of 95 (72.6%), and for the circumflex (CX) artery, 11 out of 14 (78.6%). Keon and colleagues[9] in their study of 1,718 patients reported patency rates of 73% at 1 year, 62% at 5 years, and 51% at 10 years. Qureshi and associates,[21] in a much smaller series of 278 patients, restudied 81 grafts and found a late patency rate of 89% in asymptomatic patients but only a patency rate of 58% in patients with recurrent symptoms (interval: 1 to 8 years; mean follow-up: 40 months). This demonstrated good correlation between the relief of symptoms and the patency of grafts. Throughout the reported studies in the literature, the range of patency rates for vein grafts with coronary endarterectomy is from 100% at 3 to 18 months postsurgery[16] down to 51% at 10 years after surgery.[9]

Long-Term Clinical Improvement

Symptomatic relief after endarterectomy and vein grafting does vary with surgical experiences and methods of reporting (Table 1). Livesay and associates[8] reported that 52% of their patients with endarterectomy procedures were asymptomatic at 5 years, yet 83% of their patients had a single RCA endarterectomy and only 4% had multiple endarterectomies. Brenowitz and colleagues[10] (Table 2) reported that 50% of their patients had multiple endarterectomy procedures and there was an equal number of single endarterectomies to both the left coronary artery and RCA systems. Eighty-seven percent of their patients were angina free at 1 year postsurgery, but this decreased at a rate of 6% per year. Conventional grafting was slightly better, with 71.1% of patients asymptomatic at an average follow-up of 67.8 months. Keon and associates[9] also reported on the work status of 585 patients at 5 years: 68 (12%) were unable to work, 27 (5%) were unemployed, 124 (21%) had retired, and 63% had returned to work. Amazingly, at 8 years, 128 patients were re-evaluated for work status, with 65% still working.

Table 2
Current Angina Status of 3,011 Patients
Average Follow-Up: 58.3 Months
As Reported By Brenowitz[10]

	No Angina		Angina		
	No.	Percent	Class	No.	Percent
Group A (1,575 pts; avg 67.8 mos)	1,121	71.1	I–II	382	24.3
			III–IV	72	4.6
Group B (747 pts; avg 51.4 mos)	504	67.5	I–II	208	27.8
			III–IV	35	4.7
Group C (689 pts; avg 43.9 mos)	457	66.3	I–II	204	29.6
			III–IV	28	4.1
All endarterectomy pts (1,436 pts; avg 47.8 mos)	961	66.9	I–II	412	28.7
			III–IV	63	4.4

Late Survival

As noted in Table 1, late survival rates of the three large series do not seem much different from one another at 10 and 12 years. Brenowitz et al.[10] do note a reduction in survival rates between the groups without endarterectomy (92%) and/or with only one endarterectomy (92%) and the group with multiple endarterectomies (83%). When two or more risk factors are accounted for in these same groups, the survival rates are 62%, 54%, and 37%, respectively. If severe left ventricular function (ejection fraction < 0.35) is correlated to the five-year survival for each group, the rates are 63%, 57%, and 47%, respectively. Livesay and colleagues[8] reported five-year survival rates of 90% for coronary artery bypass alone compared to 86% for coronary endarterectomy, although, as previously stated, the majority of endarterectomy procedures were to the RCA system.

Late Morphological Findings

Goldstein and associates[22] angiographically restudied 40 patients early (mean 19 days) and 27 patients in a late postoperative period (mean 19 months). Grafts to endarterectomized vessels were 90% patent (47 out of 50) for the early group but only 64% patent (27 out of 40) in the late study period. Careful attention to the appearance of the endarterectomized vessels demonstrated differences ranging from large-caliber, smooth-walled vessels to attenuated vessels with irregular walls. There was a tendency toward "shrinkage" of these vessels in the late study group, suggesting some type of fibrosis.

This has been confirmed recently in the histologically studied endarterectomized coronary arteries examined by the Ottawa Heart Institute[23] in 51 patients who died at varying intervals after coronary artery surgery with at least one endarterectomy. With specimens examined at 30 days or less, the main pathological finding was fibrin-platelet mural thrombus on the arterial wall with little tissue reaction. The striking feature at 5 years or greater was an intense myofibrointimal proliferation, including some segments without stenosis but many segments with moderate to severe stenosis. Only a few endarterectomized vessels showed atherosclerosis. Electron microscopic examination of the segments demonstrated increasing amounts of collagen and elastic fiber deposition associated with the spindle cell featuring definite characteristics of myofibrolastosis. This histologic study confirmed that fibrosis and intense proliferation of cellular elements are responsible for the late obstructive angiographic appearance much more often than atherosclerosis.

Discussion

Coronary artery endarterectomy provides an alternative, as well as an adjunct, to coronary revascularization for patients with extremely obstructive, diffuse atherosclerosis, who may otherwise be denied its benefit or subjected to incomplete revascularization or even transplantation. This procedure has controversial aspects, such as an increased mortality rate, lower graft patency, increased perioperative myocardial infarction rates, and lower survival rates compared to coronary artery bypass alone. This may, in part, be due to the procedure, but the alternative outcome of failure in bypassing the diffuse arterial lesions effectively will likely lead to adverse late cardiac events.[24,25] In the larger studies (Table 1), outcomes for this procedure are commendable. This undoubtedly reflects an increase in patients, a significant degree of technical discipline, and a commitment to this procedure when indicated.[8-10] Technically, Brenowitz et al.[10] have stressed that all atheromatous material must be removed distal to the arteriotomy site and from numerous coronary artery branches. For the LAD system, either multiple arteriotomies or a long 10 to 15 cm arteriotomy patched over by a vein graft is frequently necessary for success. Livesay et al.[8] have demonstrated a drop in operative mortality rates from 6.5% to 3.4% as years of experience were accumulated. Keon et al.[9] also indicated that major advances in cardiac surgery during the past decade, as well as increasing experience, contribute to improvement of results.

At the present time, carefully selected patients can benefit from the procedure, and, with additional advances in the future, this procedure may well be safer with improved short- and long-term benefits. For example, Keogh and colleagues[26] have used angioscopic evaluation of endarterectomy end points. Fourteen major intraluminal flaps were demonstrated at 29 visualized endpoints. The relationship between the intraluminal morphology observed at operation and patency rates needs further assessment, but angioscopy could become a valuable tool in confirming endarterectomy completeness and identifying technical problems that could cause early vessel closure and graft failure.

Another theoretically-possible, superior alternative that Mestres and associates[27] were first to report and recommend was the use of the IMA to bypass the endarterectomized LAD. This method was successfully used on five patients. Harjola and colleagues[28] reported 1 year later that 56% of the 96 endarterectomized left diagonal or LAD arteries were bypassed using the IMA. They felt that the belief that the IMA was not a suitable conduit for bypassing an endarterectomized vessel was a misconception. A prospective and randomized study is needed, but more IMA usage with endarterectomy may prevent the long-term complication of vein graft stenosis we have observed (Fig. 3). The results from the left IMA providing inflow to the long vein patch on the endarterectomized LAD (Chapter 23) could be

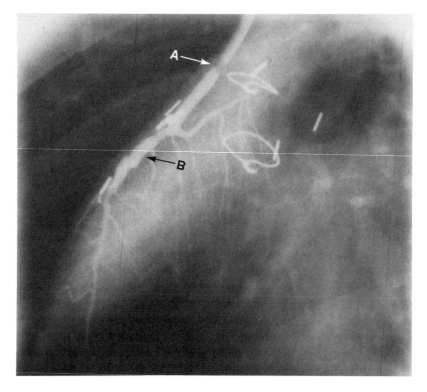

Fig. 3. Stenotic 10-year-old vein graft to an extensive endarterectomy of a left anterior descending (LAD). (A) stenosis; (B) vein patch.

compared as well. These techniques have the drawback of prolonged myocardial ischemic periods. It may be that myocardial preservation with cold-blood cardioplegia will prove its effectiveness in this situation.[11]

With a changing patient population, including the elderly, the diabetic, and those who have had multiple transluminal angioplasty procedures, diffuse coronary disease may be on the increase. This increase will necessitate procedures, such as sequential grafting, patch grafting and, for sure, endarterectomy to provide nearly complete revascularization. Each patient situation will require the selection of a particular revascularization method based on the surgeon's ability and comfort level, as well as the perceived probability that a particular procedure will likely provide immediate and lasting coronary blood flow. Extensive coronary endarterectomy will need to be thought of with increasing frequency as an alternative and/or an adjunct to other methods of revascularization, even heart transplantation.

References

1. Bailey CP, May A, Lemon NM. Survival after coronary endarterectomy in man. JAMA 1957; 164:641–646.
2. May AM. Coronary endarterectomy: curettement of coronary arteries in dogs. Am J Surg 1957; 93:969–973.
3. Longmire WP Jr, Cannon JA, Kattus AA. Direct-vision coronary endarterectomy for angina pectoris. N Engl J Med 1958; 259:993–999.
4. Sabiston DC Jr, Blalock A. Coronary thromboendarterectomy for angina pectoris. Postgrad Med 1961; 29:439–450.
5. Effler DB, Groves LK, Sones FM Jr, Shirey EK. Endarterectomy in the treatment of coronary artery disease. J Thorac Cardiovasc Surg 1964; 47:98–108.
6. Effler DB, Groves LK, Suarez EL, Favaloro RG. Direct coronary artery surgery with endarterectomy and patch graft reconstruction: clinical application and technical consideration. J Thorac Cardiovasc Surg 1967; 53:93–101.
7. Johnson WD, Brenowitz JB, Kayser LK. Surgery for diffuse coronary disease. Cardiology 1986; 4:35–38.
8. Livesay JJ, Cooley DA, Hallman GL. Early and late results of coronary endarterectomy. J Thorac Cardiovasc Surg 1986; 92:649–660.
9. Keon WJ, Masteres RG, Koshal A, Hendry P, et al. Coronary endarterectomy: an adjunct to coronary artery bypass grafting. Surg Clin North Am 1988; 68:669–678.
10. Brenowitz JB, Kayser KL, Johnson WD. Results of coronary artery endarterectomy and reconstruction. J Thorac Cardiovasc Surg 1988; 95:1–10.

11. Buckberg GD. Studies of controlled reperfusion after ischemia: a series of experimental and clinical observations from the Division of Thoracic Surgery, UCLA School of Medicine. J Thorac Cardiovasc Surg 1986; 92:483–648.

12. Sommerhaug G, Wolfe SF, Reid DA, Lindsey DE. Early clinical results of long coronary arteriotomy, endarterectomy and reconstruction combined with multiple bypass grafting for severe coronary artery disease. Am J Cardiol 1990; 66:651–659.

13. Shapiro N, Lumia FJ, Gottdiener JS, German P, et al. Adjunct endarterectomy of the left anterior descending coronary artery. Ann Thorac Surg 1988; 46:289–296.

14. Ladowski JS, Scholylien MH, Underhill DJ, Peterson AC. Endarterectomy, vein patch, and mammary bypass of the anterior descending artery. Ann Thorac Surg 1991; 52:1187–1189.

15. Hockberg MS, Merrill WH, Michelis LL. Result of combined coronary endarterectomy and coronary bypass for diffuse coronary artery disease. J Thorac Cardiovasc Surg 1978; 75:38–46.

16. Kuijpers PJ, Locquet LK, Skotnicki SH. Distal gas endarterectomy and venous bypass in coronary artery surgery. J Cardiovasc Surg (Torino) 1974; 15:158–162.

17. Dumanian AV. Endarterectomy of the branches of the left coronary artery in combination with an aorto-to-coronary artery reverse saphenous vein graft. J Cardiovasc Surg (Torino) 1974; 15:154–157.

18. Wallash E, Weinstein G, Franzene AJ, Stertzer SH. The use of distal right coronary endarterectomy and saphenous coronary bypass to decrease total grafts and extend operability in patients with coronary artery disease. In: Norman JC, ed. Coronary Artery Medicine and Surgery: Concepts and Controversies. New York: Appleton-Century-Crofts, 1975: Chap. 68.

19. Halim MB, Qureshi SA, Towers MK, Yacoub MH. Early and late results of combined endarterectomy and coronary bypass grafting for diffuse coronary disease. Am J Cardiol 1982; 49:1623–1626.

20. Miller DC, Stuison EB, Oyer PE, Reitz BP, et al. Long-term clinical assessment of the efficacy of adjunctive coronary endarterectomy. J Thorac Cardiovasc Surg 1981; 81:21–29.

21. Qureshi SA, Halim MB, Pillai R, Smith P, et al. Endarterectomy of the left coronary system: analysis of a 10 year experience. J Thorac Cardiovasc Surg 1985; 89:852–859.

22. Goldstein J, Cooper E, Saltrups A, Boxall J. Angiographic assessment of graft patency after coronary endarterectomy. J Thorac Cardiovasc Surg 1991; 102:539–545.

23. Walley VM, Byard RW, Keon WJ. A study of the sequential morphologic changes after manual coronary endarterectomy. J Thorac Caridovasc Surg 1991; 102:890–894.

24. Cukingman RA, Carey JS, Wittig JH, Brown BG. Influence of complete coronary revascularization on relief of angina. J Thorac Cardiovasc Surg 1980; 79:188–193.

25. Lawrie GM, Morris GC Jr, Silver A, Wagner WF, et al. The influence of residual disease after coronary bypass on the 5 year survival rate of 1274 men with coronary artery disease. Circulation 1982; 66:717–23.

26. Keogh BE, Bidstrup BP, Taylor KM, Sapsford RN. Angioscopic evaluation of intravascular morphology after coronary endarterectomy. Ann Thorac Surg 1991; 52:766–772.

27. Mestres CA, Iqual A, Torrents A, Esplugas E, et al. Endarterectomy of the LAD and internal mammary artery grafting. Scand J Thor Cardiovasc Surg 1987; 21:141–143.

28. Harjula PT, Harzula ALJ, Jarvinen A. Coronary bypass grafting with multiple coronary endarterectomies. Walter PJ, ed. Treatment of end-stage coronary artery disease. Adv Cardiol 1988; 36:8–12.

Chapter 25

Operative Transluminal Coronary Artery Angioplasty

Masahiro Endo

Complete revascularization during coronary artery bypass grafting (CABG) is necessary for long-term angina relief and increased longevity.[1,2] This generally can be achieved by additional grafting, endarterectomy, the sequential bypass technique, or the splitting of lesions with onlay patch grafts, but occasionally the location of the pathology and the anatomy of the coronary arteries is such that complete revascularization is difficult or impossible. Operative transluminal coronary angioplasty (OTCA) was introduced as an adjunctive method of myocardial revascularization to treat inaccessible or otherwise nonbypassable vessels rapidly during a CABG.

Dilatation of atherosclerotic lesions was first proposed by Dotter[3] in 1963. Development and refinement of Dotter's concept was slow to develop, mostly in Europe, but then in 1974, Gruntzig and Hopff[4] introduced a flexible double-lumen catheter with a coaxially mounted nondistensible balloon. By using a guidewire with fluoroscopic visualization, this balloon catheter could be positioned percutaneously for the treatment of coronary stenosis. This method revolutionized the procedure. By 1982, Wallsh et al.[5] reported the use of OTCA for stenotic lesions both proximal and distal to the planned CABG graft site. The stenoses considered were in distal branches or arteries too small for further bypass grafting. Katz et al.,[6] in 1982, expanded the indication of OTCA to multiple lesions proximal to the arterial graft

From Grooters RK and Nishida H: (editors): *Alternative Bypass Conduits and Methods for Surgical Coronary Revascularization.* © Futura Publishing Co., Inc., Armonk, NY, 1994.

site to relieve entrapped diagonal and septal branches of significant but subgraftable diameter. Other investigators[7–9] reported their experiences (Table 1), and some used various catheters and dilatation techniques (Table 2). Because of reported limitations with coaxial balloon catheters mainly due to technical difficulties and complications that occurred during catheter advancement and placement, Fogarty et al.[9] introduced the linear extrusion balloon dilatation concept (Fig. 1) and successfully dilated 19 out of 22 lesions.

The most extensive experience of OTCA is recently reported by Urschel et al.[10] with an experience of 3,197 lesions attempted in 1,000 patients with an intraoperative success rate (a 50% or greater decrease in stenotic diameter) of 67%. Postoperative angiography (1 to 7 years postoperatively) was performed on 51 patients and demon-

Table 1
Reports of OTCA Results

Author/ (Year)	OTCAs Done	Operative Success; Reported Percent	Operative Mortality (Percent)	Lesions Studies angiographically/ Results no. (%)/ time postop)
Wallsh[5]/ (1982)	77	77 dilated (100%) unsuccessful attempts ?	1 of 58 (1.7%)	24 (86.1% patency) (16<4 mo; 8–20.5 mos)
Katz[6]/ (1982)	11 (proximal to LAD graft site)	11 dilated (100%) unsuccessful attempts?	0 (0.0%)	3 (100% patency) (10 days)
Mills[7]/ (1983)	93 attempts	75 dilated (81%)	0 (0.0%)	28 of 31 patent (93%) (4.2 mos)
Roberts[8]/ (1983)	23 attempts	22 dilated (94%)	0 (0.0%)	9 of 23 improved (39%) (10 days) 4 of 12 improved (31%) (12 mo)
Forgarty[9]/ (1984)	64 attempts	54 dilated (86%)	0 (0.0%)	not done
Urschel[10]/ (1990)	3,197 attempts	2,163 dilated (67%)	19 of 1,000 (1.9%)	137 of 167 patent (82%) (1–7 yrs)
Endo/ (present)	42 attempts	33 dilated (77%)	1 of 40 (2.5%)	19 of 40 improved (47.5%) (1 mo or greater)

Table 2
Review of OTCA Techniques

Author/ (Year)	Type of Balloon (Diameter of Balloon)	Techniques of Dilatation No. of dilatations/time (sec)/pressure (atm)		
Wallsh[5]/ (1982)	coaxial (2.0–3.7 mm)	?	15	6–8 atm
Katz[6]/ (1982)	coaxial (2.0–3.0 mm)	2–4	15	sequential 4–7 atm
Mills[7]/ (1983)	coaxial (1.5–2.5 mm)	3	10	5–10 atm
	linear extrusion	3	30	7–10 atm
Roberts[8]/ (1983)	coaxial (2.0–3.7 mm)	?	15–20	up to 6 atm
Fogarty[9]/ (1984)	linear extrusion (4 mm)	?	60	hand pressure
Urschel[10]/ (1990)	coaxial (2.0–4.0 mm)	3	?	10 atm
Endo/ (present)	coaxial (size ?)	1	120	6 atm

strated that 137 out of 167 (82%) successful angioplasties were still patent. This study was designed to evaluate the effect of "competitive flow" on the bypass graft. They concluded that intraoperative balloon angioplasty had no detrimental effect on bypass graft patency, which was 84%.

We would like to share our varied, but limited, experience conducting OTCA on 42 lesions in 40 of the 1,700 patients who have undergone CABG at The Heart Institute of Japan from 1982 to 1991. Angiography was performed 1 month or more postoperatively on all except two patients. The indications for using the OTCA, selectivity considerations, and the true clinical value of the OTCA remain our concern with this adjunct and/or alternative.

Method

Coronary arteriograms of patients selected for CABG were reviewed before surgery to identify any obstructions that might prevent complete revascularization by grafting methods. Four anatomical and

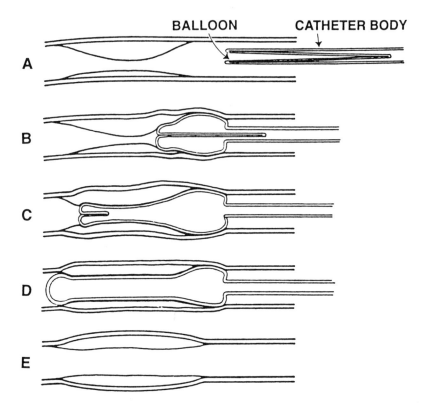

Fig. 1. Linear extrusion balloon dilatation concept. (A) Catheter is located just proximal to the stenotic segment. (B) Fluid injection results in partial extrusion. (C) Continued extrusion. (D) Balloon just prior to complete inflation. (E) Postdilation result (from Fogarty TJ et al.[9]).

pathological relationships evolved and are illustrated in Fig. 2. They include Group I—lesions in distal vessels or branches not large enough to accept a bypass conduit; Group II—a stenotic coronary artery to which no bypass graft is planned, but grafts to other coronary arteries are needed; Group III—antegrade dilatation of a left main stenosis; Group IV— a multiple stenosis proximal to the bypass conduit to revascularize an inaccessible branch such as a septal or diagonal artery; the most proximal stenosis is untreated.

Postoperative angiographic determinations were planned for all patients 1 month or more after CABG and were categorized as (1)

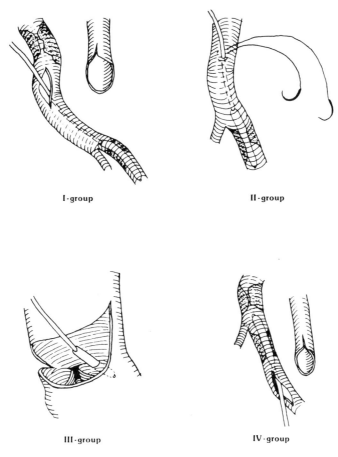

Fig. 2. Methods of Operative Transluminal Coronary Angioplasty (OTCA). Coaxial systems are used over a guidewire if needed. Group I: distal lesions; Group II: dilating distal lesions without proximal grafting; Group III: antegrade dilation of left main trunk; Group IV: retrograde dilation of tandem lesion proximal to the graft site.

success—a regression of the dilated lesion greater than 20%; (2) unchanged—the stenosis remains within ± 20% of its preoperative determination; (3) progression—a 20% or more increase in the stenosis compared to its preoperative determination; and (4) technical failure—a rupture or perforation of the coronary arteries.

Technique

The fixed guidewire coaxial systems made by USCI (division of C.R. Bard, Inc., Murray Hill, NJ) and SciMed Life Systems (Minneapolis, Minn) were selected for our OTCA procedures. Except for the left main lesion treated through the aortotomy, all procedures were performed through a coronary arteriotomy. Each stenotic lesion was assessed with Parsonnet dilator probes (C.R. Bard, Inc.) to target the lesion distance and determine intraluminal coronary artery size. The OTCA catheter was then inserted and positioned through the lesion to be dilated. Its position was generally easy to confirm by direct vision or light-touch palpation. The balloon catheter was gradually inflated by using saline in the inflation device Indeflator from Advanced Cardiovascular Systems, Inc. (Santa Clara, Calif) to generate six atmospheres of pressure for 2 minutes. After the OTCA was complete, soft plastic tubing, 3 French in diameter, was inserted through the arteriotomy and the dilated lesion. Then any loosened atherosclerotic debris was flushed with a cardioplegia solution. The dilated lesion was again probed and considered successful if a probe (usually 1.5 mm or greater) would pass through the lesion. The bypass grafting was then conducted.

Results

Of the 1,700 patients receiving CABG at The Heart Institute of Japan from 1982 to 1991, OTCA was concomitantly performed on 40 patients (33 males, 7 females) with an age range of 7 to 74 years. One death occurred (2.5%). This occurred in a seven-year-old boy with preexisting cardiogenic shock prior to surgery from which he did not recover. A perioperative myocardial infarction confirmed by elevated enzymes and electrocardiographic changes occurred in one patient (2.5%). Graft patency was angiographically determined in all patients, except the surgical death in one patient with postoperative hepatitis. Of the 77 grafts studied (38 patients), 72 grafts were patent (93.5%). Thirty-two of the 42 lesions (77.5%) attempted were considered an intraoperative success. Angiographic follow-up 1 month or more postoperatively confirmed an overall success rate of 47.5%, but the rate was different for each group (Table 3). All surviving patients were asymptomatic at follow-up, including the three patients with patent, dilated stenosis but closed vein grafts to the same artery.

Table 3
Results of Operative Transluminal Coronary Angioplasty

	Group 1	Group 2	Group 3	Group 4	Total Groups
Lesion Success	8 (38%)	7 (54%)	1 (100%)	3 (60%)	19 (47.5%)
Unchanged	6 (29%)	3 (23%)	0	0	9 (22.5%)
Progression	3 (14%)	0	0	0	3 (7.5%)
Unpassed (failure)	4 (19%)	3 (23%)	0	2 (40%)	9 (22.5%)
Unknown (without postoperative angiogram)	1 (hepatitis)	0	0	1(death)	2

Case Reports

Case 1: male, age 64(Fig. 3)

The patient had an old inferior myocardial infarction with angina. A 90% stenosis of the proximal left anterior descending (LAD) and a 99% stenosis of the proximal right coronary artery (RCA) with a distal 75% stenosis was confirmed angiographically. An OTCA was performed on the distal RCA stenosis, and a double CABG was performed. The 75% stenosis decreased angiographically to a 20% stenosis, and the patency of both grafts was observed.

Case 2: male, age 62 (Fig. 4)

This patient was admitted for unstable angina. A left main stenosis (75%), a 99% stenosis of the proximal LAD, and a proximal 90% stenosis of a very small (hypoplastic) RCA was diagnosed. Double CABG was performed to the LAD and the left circumflex (CX) artery. A tiny arteriotomy was made in the normal RCA and was closed after OTCA without grafting. The patency of both grafts was observed, and the stenosis of the RCA decreased to 25%.

Case 3: female, age 19 (Fig. 5)

The patient experienced unstable angina due to an aortitis syndrome. A 99% stenosis of the left main trunk was confirmed. After an

PREOPERATION   **POSTOPERATION**

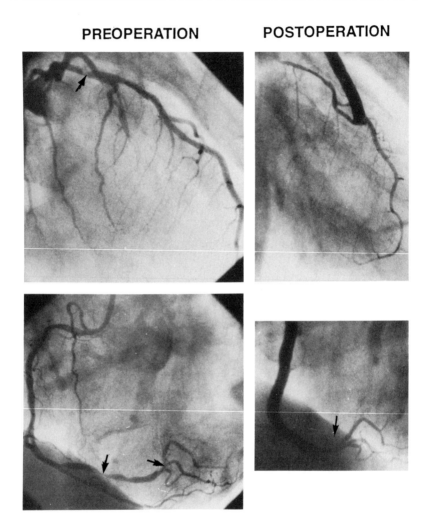

Fig. 3. Case 1. OTCA was performed for the distal stenosis of the right coronary artery (RCA). Note the improvement in the lower right-hand photo.

aortotomy, 0.5 and 1.0 mm probes were used to identify and dilate the left main ostium. Subsequently, an OTCA was performed with 2.0 and 2.5 mm balloon catheters. As tension was applied to the 2.5 mm balloon during its inflation, an endarterectomy of the ostial intima was performed with a fine knife. Disappearance of the left main lesion was observed on the postoperative angiogram, and collateral vessels from the RCA had also disappeared.

PRE OPERATION

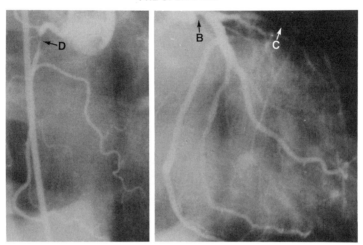

POST OPERATION

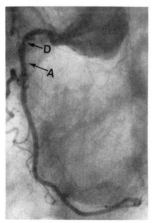

Fig. 4. Case 2. Dilatation representative of the Group II method. No graft used. Note the improvement from 90% stenosis to residual 25% stenosis (labeled D). (A) RCA. (B) left main lesion. (C) left anterior descending lesion.(D) RCA lesion improved.

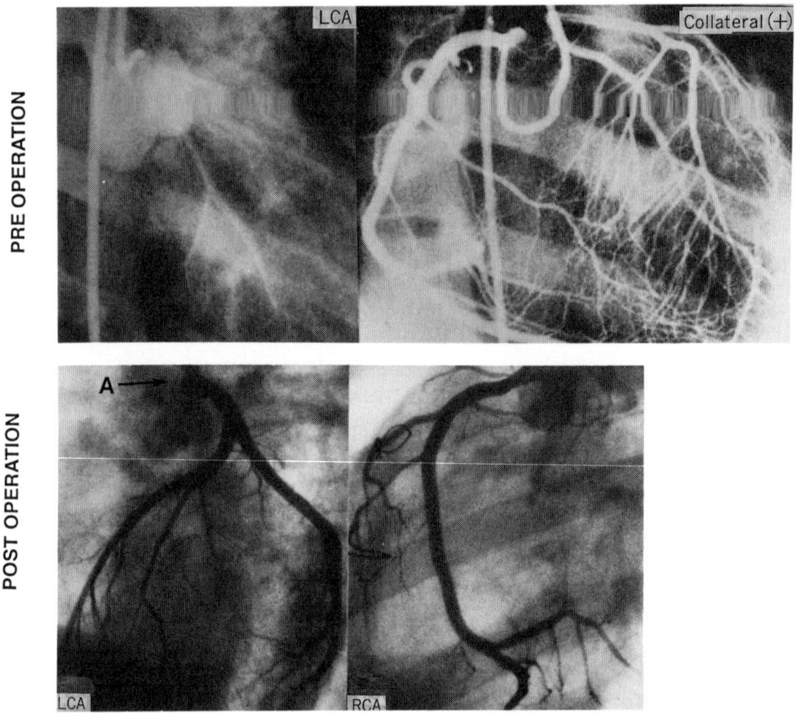

Fig. 5. Case 3. 100% left main obstruction collateralized from the RCA (A) After an OTCA, the left main ostium appeared normal (lower left photo).

Discussion

OTCA has an appeal as an adjunct with CABG and in highly selective situations may be an alternative. The techniques appear safe, and the equipment (coaxial or extrusion) is easy to use. Catheter manipulation can be performed rapidly, adding no more than a few minutes of crossclamp time. Coronary stenosis and intraoperative results of dilatation can be assessed quickly by graduated probes, but the only true test of the procedure's ability to provide an adequate channel to the runoff vascular bed is the short- and long-term angiography. Encouraging results were first reported by Wallsh et al.[5] Thirty-four coronary artery stenoses distal to the insertion of the saphenous vein graft (SVG) were dilated. Of the 15 dilated lesions studied with postoperative angiography, 12 lesions (80%) showed a significant increase in diameter. Other investigators[7-10] obtained variable results but with a variety of equipment and methods of dilatation (Table 2).

At first glance, our angiographic success rate of 47.5% appears inferior to the other studies.[5-7] This conclusion may, in part, be due to (1) different postoperative angiographic schedules; (2) the mixtures of lesions selected; (3) an oriental population with smaller coronary anatomies; and (4) probably different techniques. Until all these factors are standardized, the true meaning of the data reported on this procedure will remain clouded.

Adding an OTCA to the bypass procedure does not increase operative mortality or the perioperative myocardial infarction rate, but we, like Roberts et al.[8] are concerned about the discrepancy between symptomatic relief and angiographic improvement in the surviving patients. Most patients are relieved of their angina (92%), but less than a majority of these (33%) had improvement in the angiographic appearance of the dilated stenosis. This procedure was introduced because of concerns about the adverse effects that Jones and coworkers documented[1] on long-term survival and symptom relief following incomplete coronary revascularization. This work may not be an applicable reason for the use of an OTCA. The CABG today is certainly more complete, and surgeons have more time for complete revascularization because of improved myocardial preservation techniques in locating difficult vessels and treating diffusely diseased vessels with endarterectomy or multiple bypasses.

The event of bypass graft closure associated with an OTCA of a proximal lesion is somewhat disturbing. This raises the concern as to whether it is better for the patient to have a vessel dependent on a diseased proximal segment (though patent) or a normal patent graft. We realize that Urschel and his colleagues,[10] from their observation, believe that competitive flow is not a major problem, but we have observed three patients with occluded vein grafts to vessels with previously dilated lesions now patent but stenotic. Maybe the graft would have been patent if the conduit had been an internal mammary artery (IMA). Nonetheless, we are still cautious about choosing which proximal pathology to treat with an OTCA.

In conclusion, despite the findings of previous studies, we have to raise questions about this procedure's efficacy. Questioning the amount of value added to the CABG by doing an OTCA, although difficult to measure, is necessary. An objective determination of an OTCA's overall effect compared to that of alternative modes of therapy will need further prospective study, or else, this part of the surgeon's armamentarium, though a quick and safe adjunct and/or alternative, will remain dubious.

References

1. Jones El, Craver JM, King SB, Douglas JS, et al. Clinical, anatomic and functional descriptors influencing morbidity, survival and adequacy of revascularization following coronary bypass. Ann Surg 1980; 192: 390–402.
2. Buda AJ, MacDonald IL, Anderson MJ, Strauss HD, et al. Long-term results following coronary bypass operation: importance of preoperative factors and complete revascularization. J Thorac Cardiovasc Surg 1981; 82:383–390.
3. Dotter CT. Cardiac catheterization and angiographic techniques of the future. Cesk Radiol 1965; 19:217–223.
4. Gruntzig A, Hopff H. Perkutane rekanalisation chronischer arterieller verschlusse mit einem neuen dilatationskatheter. Dtsch Med Wochenschr 1974; 99:2503–2509.
5. Wallsh E, Franzone AJ, Weinstein GS, Alean K, et al. Use of operative transluminal coronary angioplasty as an adjunct to coronary artery bypass. J Thorac Cardiovasc Surg 1982; 84:843–848.
6. Katz RJ, Leiboff RH, Aaron BL, Mills M, et al. Intraoperative retrograde balloon angioplasty of the left anterior descending coronary artery for reperfusion of jeopardized proximal branches. Circulation 1982; 66(suppl. I):I-30–I-34.
7. Mills NL, Doyle DP, Kalchoff WP. Technique and results of operative transluminal angioplasty in 81 consecutive patients. J Thorac Cardiovasc Surg 1983; 86:689–696.
8. Roberts AJ, Faro RS, Feldman RL, Conti CR, et al. Comparison of early and long-term results with intraoperative transluminal balloon catheter dilatation and coronary artery bypass grafting. J Thorac Cardiovasc Surg 1983; 86:435–440.
9. Fogarty TJ, Kinney TB. Intraoperative coronary artery balloon catheter dilatation. Am Heart J 1984; 107:845–851.
10. Urschel HC Jr, Razzuk MA, Miller E, Chung SY. Operative transluminal balloon angioplasty. J Thorac Cardiovasc Surg 1990; 99:581–589.

Chapter 26

Operative Transluminal Laser Coronary Angioplasty

Masahiro Endo

Transluminal laser irradiation as a potential treatment of coronary atherosclerosis was not investigated intensively until Choy et al.,[1] Macruz et al.,[2] and Lee et al.[3] demonstrated plaque ablation using argon laser energy transmitted through optical fibers. This was promising, but Abela and coworkers[4] studied and found three types of laser energy (carbon dioxide, Nd-YAG, and argon) that could cut a remarkably clean channel, but there were additional and undesirable adjacent zones of thermal and acoustic injury discovered in the targeted tissue. Precise parameters and control of the energy was needed to prevent unwanted normal arterial wall injury or perforation.[4-6] Nonetheless, the laser seemed very appropriate for treating stenosis of femoral and popliteal arteries,[7,8] particularly when balloon angioplasty was added to enlarge the channels to provide better blood flow and, thus, prevent thrombosis.[9] A spherical metal lip ("hot tip") was added to the end of the laser fiber to concentrate the energy.[10] This enlarged the channel and could be used for larger arteries.

Choy and coworkers[11] were the first to clinically apply the laser to coronary arteries. Operative transluminal laser coronary angioplasty (OTLCA) successfully relieved seven of eight proximal stenoses prior to bypass grafting of the vessel lased, but subsequently, angiography demonstrated occlusion of all the treated le-

From Grooters RK and Nishida H: (editors): *Alternative Bypass Conduits and Methods for Surgical Coronary Revascularization.* © Futura Publishing Co., Inc., Armonk, NY, 1994.

sions. These small, new channels most likely occluded secondary to competitive flow. By 1985, Livesay and colleagues[12] reported their initial results of "laser endarterectomy" using a hand-held CO_2 laser fitted with a 1.5-mm outer-diameter hollow waveguide (Fig. 1). Once

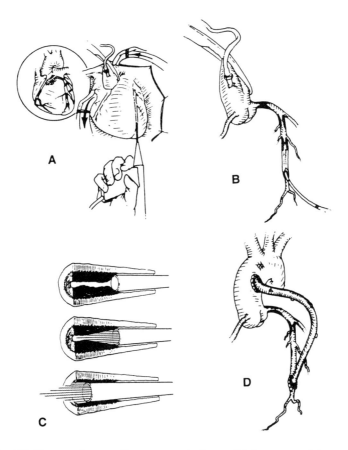

Fig. 1. (A) Proposed operative approach to multiple segmental coronary stenosis using the hand-held CO_2 laser (reported by Livesay et al.[12]). (B) Calibrated coronary probes for assessing the location and severity of segmental coronary stenosis. (C) Laser coronary endarterectomy relieves coronary stenosis. Each laser impulse cuts a conical opening in the plaque. (Multiple, short impulses are desired to prevent thermal injury to the artery.) (D) Aortocoronary bypass completes revascularization after laser coronary endarterectomy opens additional tributaries and runoff. (Reprinted with permission from the Texas Heart Institute Journal 1984; 11:278).

the laser was aligned with the vessel, a series of laser pulses were begun until the plaque was penetrated. The size of the lumen was assessed by probes, and the target was inspected by an angioscope. The vessel was flushed with cardioplegia to remove debris, and a graft was sutured to the arteriotomy. Operative success was achieved in 15 out of 16 coronary stenoses, and follow-up angiography demonstrated a 75% patency rate. In a subsequent report,[13] operative success was noted in 37 out of 40 diseased vessels, with tandem stenosis of lesions peripheral to the graft. The patency rate confirmed by angiography 1 week to 6 months after surgery remained the same (76%).

During this same period of time, Sanborn et al.,[14] Cumberland et al.,[15] and Crea et al.[16] performed percutaneous transluminal coronary laser angioplasty during cardiac catheterization. The 1.7 mm argon laser probe was threaded over a guidewire for control. There were a few good results, but there were high complication rates of perforation and myocardial infarction.

More recently, Litvack and coworkers[17] have successfully used the excimer laser percutaneously to ablate vein graft stenoses in two patients. The intraoperative use of the excimer laser has recently been reported by Olliver and colleagues[18] on ten patients. The ultraviolet-tipped fiberoptic scope (Fig. 2) was introduced upstream from the arteriotomy in seven patients and downstream in three patients. All recanalized segments, except one, were patent when studied angiographically at 6 months. The one patient not studied died of a perioperative myocardial infarction. Microscopic examination of the artery treated with the excimer laser showed a fracture of the atherosclerotic material at the periphery of the area treated, resulting in an

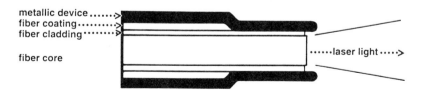

Fig. 2. Diagram of the fiber tip. A metallic device is fitted to the distal extremity of the fiber to prevent mechanical injury of the endothelium during intraluminal manipulation and to avoid any fiber core rupture while ablation is going on. This metal tip lets all the laser light flow free without heating under UV radiation. When the device is in contact with the plaque, the fiber core is about 0.5 mm from the surface of the tissue (from Ollivier JP, et al.[17]).

area of intimal hemorrhage. Manipulation of the fiberoptic instrument may have contributed to this fracture but was not considered the cause of death. It is hoped that the ultraviolet (UV) photo ablative process from the excimer laser is less destructive to the neighboring tissue than is the thermal energy of the CO_2, argon, or Nd-YAG lasers. We have begun our OTLCA investigation by trying to compare the usage of Nd-YAG laser and excimer laser energy in the clinical and operative setting. So far, eight lesions in six patients have been treated with these two alternatives.

Methods

The lesions to be lased are chosen preoperatively from angiographic evaluation and seem divisible into four classifications: (1) antegrade from the coronary arteriotomy to the distal coronary artery lesion; (2) retrograde from the coronary arteriotomy to the proximal coronary artery stenosis; (3) through an aortotomy (transaortic approach) antegrade from the coronary ostium to a distal lesion; and (4) direct antegrade approach through a vein graft incision on a vein graft stenosis. One month after surgery, all survivors will undergo coronary angiographic studies to determine patency rates and lesion reduction.

Operative Technique

After extracorporeal circulation is instituted using moderate hypothermia (28°C), myocardial preservation is accomplished with a cold (4°C) potassium cardioplegia solution. The coronary arteries to be bypassed or lased and old vein grafts to be lased are exposed by dissection, and the plaque (distal or proximal) is identified by palpation and inspection. The arteriotomy or venotomy is made at a location close to the lesion, if possible. If the transaortic approach is to be used, the bypass grafts are done first. Intraluminal probes are used to confirm the location of the lesion and size of the coronary artery. The amount of laser energy selected is usually 10 watts for the Nd-YAG laser and 35mJ/mm^2 for the excimer laser. The direct contact method is generally considered for the transaortic approach for the very proximal left main lesion, and an over-the-wire method is used for the lasing procedures through the coronary arteriotomy. Once the lasing is complete, intraluminal probes are used to confirm the diameter of the lesion treated. This diameter is usually 1.5 mm. Then the arteriotomy site is grafted, or the venotomy or aortotomy is closed. Cardioplegia is given after each laser procedure to identify any perforation and also, before the graft is sutured, to flush the lasered artery. Additional balloon dilatation is used if the laser-treated lesion remains stenotic as determined by intraluminal probing.

Results

Eight laser procedures were performed in six patients. There were no deaths. Nine bypass grafts were made in these six patients. Six lesions (75%) were successfully treated, of which two had adjunctive balloon angioplasty. The mean value of the stenosis determined angiographically dropped from 90.7% preprocedure to 22.5% after the procedure. One perforation was encountered using the hot-tip Nd-YAG catheter on a left main stenosis. The curvature of the left main trunk was too acute and probably should not have been used. This was repaired without incident. In another patient, the wire passed through the hard calcified lesion, but the YAG laser catheter failed to penetrate the lesion.

Case Example

A 70-year-old male with left main stenosis and severe triple vessel disease had undergone coronary artery bypass grafting 6 years before. Angiography revealed complete occlusion of the grafts to the right coronary artery (RCA) and the left anterior descending (LAD) artery. The vein graft to the circumflex (CX) artery contained a localized 90% stenosis. A double bypass using the left internal mammary artery (IMA) to the LAD and the right gastroepiploic artery (RGEA) to the posterior descending (PD) artery was accomplished. A tiny incision proximal to the lesion in the vein graft to the CX was then made. An over-the-wire laser catheter for the Holmium YAG laser was inserted, and 2.5 watts were used to ablate the lesion (Fig. 3). Postoperative angiography revealed both grafts to be patent, and the stenosis of the old graft had completely disappeared (Fig. 4).

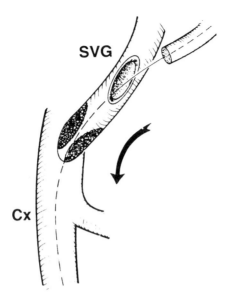

Cx: Left Coronary Circumflex Artery

Fig. 3. Lasing of the vein graft stenosis of the graft to the circumflex (CX) coronary artery.

Discussion

Incomplete revascularization is definitely a factor of early post-operative death, failure of symptom relief, and reoperation.[19] As many as 5% of patients cannot benefit completely from coronary artery bypass grafting (CABG) because of extensive disease, small artery atherosclerosis, or extremely calcified coronary artery lesions.[20] Manual endarterectomy has been performed in many of these nearly hopeless patients with a high operative mortality rate of 10%,[21] with the survivors showing symptomatic relief. The question is, will laser ablation, percutaneous or intraoperatively, be a future development with any measurable benefit or added value in assisting surgeons with these difficult patients? And if laser ablation can be beneficial, in which patients and situations should it be used?

The laser seems quick, easy, and able to open atherosclerotic lesions. The work by Livesay and coworkers[6,12] with the CO_2 laser may still hold potential that is undeveloped. Although it looks promising,

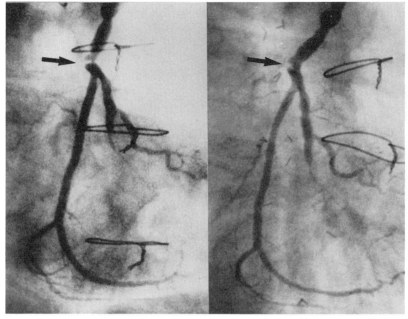

post OTLCA(Ho–YAG)

SVG: Saphenous Vein Graft

OTLCA: OperativeTransluminal Laser Coronary Angioplasty

Fig. 4. Postoperative angiogram (6 weeks) with complete ablation of the vein graft stenosis.

there is evidence to suggest increased thrombotic potential in the early postoperative period when compared to the manual endarterectomy.[22] Also, CO_2 laser energy penetrates only 2 or 3 mm and needs a dry-air environment, but argon or Nd-YAG laser energy can penetrate deeper and be used in blood or a liquid medium. The argon and Nd-YAG laser energy is attractive because optical flexible fibers can be used to transfer this energy to the targeted lesion, but exact methods are still undetermined. The excimer laser has the specific property of "cool energy" and, thus, the risk of perforation seen with thermal energy from the argon and Nd-YAG lasers is less likely. This has been demonstrated in a previous study[23] using laser angioplasty in human cadaver coronary material. Thermal laser energy was shown to have 30 times the risk of producing perforation than the excimer laser.

We have had limited experience with the excimer laser, but it is our impression that this energy source may provide the safety we need to treat coronary artery lesions. In conclusion, clinical indications for intraoperative laser usage need to be delineated based on angiographic and clinical outcomes before OTLCA is demonstrated to be a useful adjunct to coronary bypass grafting or an alternative to other methods of coronary revascularization.

References

1. Choy DSJ, Stertzer SH, Rotterdam HZ, Bruno MS. Laser coronary angioplasty: experience with 9 cadaver hearts. Am J Cardiol 1982; 50: 1209–1211.
2. Macruz R, Martins JRM, Tupinamba A, et al. Therapeutic possibilities of laser beams in atheromas. Arq Bras Cardiol 1980; 34:9–12.
3. Lee G, Ikeda RM, Kozina J, Mason DT. Laser dissolution of coronary atherosclerotic obstruction. Am Heart J 1981; 102:1074–1075.
4. Abela GS, Normann S, Cohen D, Feldman RL, et al. Effects of carbon dioxide, Nd-YAG, and argon laser radiation on coronary atheromatous plaques. Am J Cardiol 1982; 50:1198–1205.
5. Grundfest WS, Litvack F, Forrester JS, Goldenberg TSVI, et al. Laser ablation of human atherosclerotic plaque without adjacent tissue injury. J Am Coll Cardiol 1985; 5:929–933.
6. Livesay JJ, Johansen WE, Sutter LV, et al. Experimental technique of laser coronary endarterectomy and its immediate effects on atherosclerotic plaques in cadaver hearts. Tex Heart Inst J 1984; 11:280–285.
7. Ginsburg R, Kim DS, Guthaner D. Salvage of an ischemic limb by laser angioplasty: description of a new technique. Clin Cardiol 1984; 7:54–58.
8. Abela GS, Seeger JM, Barbieri E, Frazini D, et al. Laser angioplasty with angioscopic guidance in humans. J Am Coll Cardiol 1986; 8:184–192.
9. Cumberland DC, Sanborn TA, Taylor DI, Moore DJ, et al. Percutaneous laser thermal angioplasty: initial clinical results with a laser probe in total peripheral artery occlusions. Lancet 1986; 1:1457.
10. Sanborn TA, Faxon DP, Howelenschild CC, Ryan TJ. Experimental angioplasty: circumferential distribution of laser thermal energy with a laser probe. J Am Coll Cardiol 1985; 5:934–938.
11. Choy DSJ, Stertzer SH, Myler RK. Human coronary laser recanalization. Clin Cardiol 1984; 7:377–381.
12. Livesay JJ, Leachman DR, Hogan PJ, Cogsec JR, et al. Preliminary report on laser coronary endarterectomy in patients. Circulation 1985; (suppl.III)72:302.
13. Livesay JJ. Intraoperative laser coronary angioplasty. Thorac Cardiovasc Surg 1988; 35(special issue):150–154.

14. Sanborn TA, Faxon DP, Kellet MA. Percutaneous coronary laser thermal angioplasty. J Am Coll Cardiol 1986; 8:1437–1440.
15. Cumberland DC, Starkey IR, Oakley GDG, Fleming JS, et al. Percutaneous laser-assisted coronary angioplasty. Lancet 1986; 2:214.
16. Crea F, Davies G, McKenna W, Pashazade M, et al. Percutaneous laser recanalization of coronary arteries. Lancet 1986; 2:214–215.
17. Litvack F, Grundfest WS, Goldenberg TSVI, Laudenslager J, et al. Percutaneous excimer laser angioplasty of aortocoronary saphenous vein grafts. J Am Coll Cardiol 1989; 14:803–808.
18. Olliver JP, Gandjbakhch I, Avrillier S, Delettre E, et al. Intraoperative coronary artery endarterectomy with excimer laser. J Thorac Cardiovasc Surg 1990; 100:606–611.
19. Jones EL, Craver JM, King SB, Douglas JS, et al. Clinical, anatomic, and functional descriptors influencing morbidity, survival, and adequacy of revascularization following coronary bypass. Ann Surg 1980; 192:390–402.
20. CASS Principal Investigators and their Associates. Coronary artery surgery study: a randomized trial of coronary artery bypass surgery-survival data. Circulation 1983; 68:939–950.
21. Brenowitz JB, Kayser KL, Johnson WD. Results of coronary endarterectomy and reconstruction. J Thorac Cardiovasc Surg 1988; 95:1–10.
22. McVicker JH, Day AL, Savage DF, Abela GS, et al. Laser endarterectomy: a comparison of thrombotic potential following CO_2 laser vs. surgical endarterectomy. Stroke 1986; 17:266–270.
23. Ollivier JP, Avrillier S, Rougier J. Appert des lasers a excimeres a l'angioplastie coronaire. Arch Mal Coeur 1988; 81:261–265.

Part VII
Artificial Grafts in the Coronary Position

Chapter 27

The Past, Present, and Future of Small Diameter Grafts

Jonathan D. Gates and K. Craig Kent

In 1989, more than 250,000 coronary artery bypass graftings (CABG) and more than 100,000 infrainguinal arterial reconstructions were performed in the United States. The internal mammary artery (IMA) has become the gold standard for the CABG (Chapter 1), and the saphenous vein (SV) is a second standard (Chapter 2) for small vessel arterial replacement. Five-year patency rates as high as 80% have been reported when the SV is used for peripheral bypass,[1,2] and ten-year patency rates of 77% with usage of the SV are reported for CABG.[3] Although these results are admirable, there is room for improvement. Even in the best of series, 20% of vein grafts fail as a result of technical misadventure, intimal hyperplasia, or recurrent atherosclerosis. Not infrequently, the SV is too small, varicose, phlebitic, or absent. In such cases, a suitable alternative is required.[4,5]

The ideal prosthetic vascular graft has been defined but remains elusive.[6] This graft must demonstrate good handling properties and be easy to suture. It should be nonreactive, resistant to infection, and durable. Most important, the ideal conduit must be nonthrombogenic.

This quest for the ideal artificial graft has led to the development of a variety of synthetic conduits, heterografts, and homografts. Unfortunately, none of these grafts has achieved patencies that supersede or even equal that of the IMA or even the SV. Although much

From Grooters RK and Nishida H: (editors): *Alternative Bypass Conduits and Methods for Surgical Coronary Revascularization.* © Futura Publishing Co., Inc., Armonk, NY, 1994.

progress has been made, the need for a less thrombogenic small-diameter vascular graft still exists. Included in this chapter is a description of currently available vascular grafts, a discussion of the causes and mechanisms of graft failure, and a review of a variety of new approaches to small vessel bypass.

Currently Available Synthetic and Biological Grafts

The development of prosthetic bypass grafts began in the early 1950s. Initially, tubes made of Vinyon-"N" cloth were used to bridge arterial defects in dogs.[7] This was followed by the introduction of Dacron and then Teflon in 1957.[8] Matsumoto et al.[9] demonstrated acceptable patency rates in dogs using polytetrafluoroethylene (PTFE) grafts as small arterial substitutes. Campbell and associates,[10,11] in the mid 1970s, were the first to use PTFE for femoropopliteal reconstruction in humans. Today, Dacron and PTFE grafts are often used for small vessel reconstructions when autogenous grafts are not available.

Polytetrafluoroethylene (PTFE)

Polytetrafluorethylene (PTFE) is a chemically inert polymer composed of carbon and fluorine. The expanded form is derived via a mechanical stretching process that creates solid nodes connected by fine fibrils. Fibril length is the distance between nodes of PTFE (usually 28–42 microns) and determines the degree of porosity of the graft material. Aneurysm formation in early PTFE grafts was eliminated by reinforcement of the grafts with an outer circumferential layer.[12]

PTFE is available for use in humans in sizes of 3 to 20 mm and has been used as a large vessel replacement, as well as a small vessel substitute.

Dacron

Dacron is a multifilament yarn. Textile machinery usually imparts elasticity and softness to the yarn, which improves handling characteristics. Early investigators felt that the mesh characteristics of a fabric prosthesis would allow ingrowth of host tissues and promote the healing process. The yarn may be knitted, woven, or fashioned into a velour configuration. Tightly woven prostheses are minimally porous and do not require preclotting. However, these grafts are non-compliant, and handling characteristics are poor. Knitted grafts are more porous and, therefore, require preclotting; yet, they are easier to handle and suture and become more incorporated by the surrounding tissues. Dacron is employed most often as an arterial substitute for the thoracic and abdominal aorta and may also be used for extraanatomical bypasses, femoropopliteal bypasses, and, occasionally, for aortocoronary bypasses.

Heterografts

Since the pioneering work by Gross and associates[13] in 1948, heterografts from dogs,[14] sheep,[14,15] and cattle[16] have been used for arterial replacement in humans. This biological graft is created by removing nonessential proteins, via enzymatic digestion or aldehyde tanning, which diminishes the inherent antigenicity of the donor tissue. Treatments with dialdehyde starch, polyacrolein, and glutaraldehyde have all been used to create these grafts. The resulting collagenous tube incites a fibroblastic host response, yet the original structural fibers remain identifiable many years later. Heterografts were used for the femoropopliteal bypass at one time. More recently, heterografts have been used for the aortocoronary bypass.[16,17] Homografts created from human umbilical veins have also been employed for both the femoropopliteal and aortocoronary bypass.

Synthetic Grafts (Used in Peripheral Vascular Surgery)

PTFE femoropopliteal bypass grafts achieve acceptable early patency rates, but, by 5 years, a significant number of these grafts will have occluded.[18–21] Although a recent report from UCLA touted a five-year patency of 60% for all PTFE femoropopliteal bypasses,[22] other groups have found patencies to be as low as 22%.[23] A number of studies are now available, and five-year patencies average approximately 40%.[19,20]

In some reports, PTFE grafts anastomosed to the above-knee popliteal artery have been shown to be more durable when compared to those grafts placed to the below-knee popliteal artery. Those investigators reporting high patency rates for above-knee femoropopliteal bypasses advocate the preferential use of PTFE, even when the SV is available.[22] This allows preservation of the SV for a future aortocoronary bypass or a subsequent, more distal bypass in the same extremity. Although the merit of a "vein sparing" approach is debated, the above-knee femoropopliteal bypass with PTFE is certainly an excellent alternative when SV is not available.[23]

Dacron may be used for the femoropopliteal bypass, yielding five- and ten-year patency rates that are comparable to PTFE.[24] A recent retrospective review of above- and below-knee reconstructions showed the overall five-year patency rate for Dacron and PTFE to be 48% and 27%, respectively.[25] The overwhelming popularity of PTFE compared to Dacron may be related to its seemingly repellent and nonthrombogenic surface and a more aggressive marketing approach by the makers of PTFE. To date, there is no conclusive evidence that PTFE is superior to Dacron for the femoropopliteal bypass.

The patency of the prosthetic bypass to the infrapopliteal vasculature (the tibial, peroneal, and pedal vessels) is markedly reduced.[21] Whittemore et al.[20] found that only 12% of infrapopliteal bypasses with PTFE remained patent after 2 years. Quinones-Baldrich et al.[22] reported only slightly better results (three-year primary patency of 20%) with a PTFE bypass to the tibial and peroneal vessels. Autogenous conduits, such as the cephalic and lesser SV, should be the first alternative for the femorotibial bypass if the SV is not available. Synthetic grafts may be occasionally used for the infrageniculate bypass in patients with limb-threatening ischemia, when autogenous tissue is not available. Although these grafts have a limited life span, a painful ulcer or forefoot amputation may heal before the graft occludes, leaving a viable limb despite graft thrombosis.

Prosthetic grafts have been used in the extraanatomical position as femorofemoral and axillofemoral bypasses. Five-year patency rates for either of these reconstructions with PTFE or Dacron range from 60%–80%.[26–30]

Biological Grafts (Used in Peripheral Vascular Surgery)

Bovine heterografts have been used for the femoropopliteal bypass, yielding a dismal three-year patency rate of 40%.[31] Aneurysmal degeneration in a significant number of these grafts eventually led to discontinuation of their use.[32] Recently, there has been renewed interest in heterografts, but the results are still discouraging. Wagner et al.[33] reported a two-year secondary patency of 62% when the femoropopliteal bypass was performed with a series of bovine carotid heterografts.

Synthetic Grafts (Used in the Aortocoronary Bypass)

In the mid-1970s, Cohn and Collins[34] performed experimental work in dogs using 3-mm PTFE aortocoronary grafts. Unfortunately, even the short-term patency of these grafts was low.

Periodically, surgeons, when faced in their clinical practices with an inadequate SV or IMA, have used PTFE grafts for CABG. Although grafts have remained patent for up to 53 months,[35] the overall results with the prosthetic aortocoronary bypass in humans are poor (Table 1).[36–40] Although a significant number of grafts remain open for the first 2 months, graft failure then occurs at a relatively rapid pace. At least experimentally, antiplatelet therapy in dogs promotes patency of synthetic aortocoronary grafts. However, there is little definitive data available for humans that suggests that antiplatelet therapy will substantially increase patency.[41]

For a number of years, Dacron grafts have been sporadically used for CABG. Several investigators have successfully used short 3.5-mm grafts to bypass from the aorta to the proximal coronary arteries in situations where the aorta is primarily diseased. There have been few attempts to bypass atherosclerotic coronary artery disease with Dacron.[42]

Table 1
Patency of PTFE Grafts Used for Aortocoronary Artery Bypass

Author (Year)	No. of Prosthetic Grafts	Time Interval (Months)	Patency of Grafts Studied
Yokoyama[36] (1978)	5	3–6	80%
Sapsford[37] (1981)	27	3	61%
		12–24	67%
Hehrlein[38] (1984)	22	1–26	59%
Chard[39] (1987)	28	12	64%
		24	14%
Hartman[40] (1991)	2	3	100%

It has been speculated that the patency of prosthetic grafts may be higher when these grafts are used to bypass the right coronary artery (RCA). In the RCA, the flow is continuous and augmented during diastole as opposed to the left coronary artery (LCA) where flow stops in systole and occurs mostly during diastole.

Currently, PTFE should be used for the aortocoronary bypass only in urgent situations in which there is a lack of a suitable autogenous conduit. Heart transplantation in appropriate individuals should also be considered before the use of PTFE coronary artery grafting.

Biological Grafts (Used in the Aortocoronary Bypass)

The continued search for an acceptable arterial substitute to be used for the aortocoronary bypass has led to the investigation of several types of heterografts. Tomizawa et al.[15] used sheep carotid arteries treated with polyepoxy compounds for the aortocoronary bypass in dogs. Only 50% of these conduits were patent after a brief observation period of 17 days. An isolated report in 1975 described the use of two sheep carotid arterial heterografts for CABG in a man.[14] Repeat angiography 6 months postoperatively verified occlusion of both grafts.

A new heterograft receiving recent recognition is the bovine internal mammary artery conduit (BIMA), which is available in 3 to 5 mm internal diameters. Several investigators have implanted this graft in the absence of a suitable greater SV.[16,17,43,44] Recently, Suma et al.[17] used the BIMA graft for CABG in 20 patients, bypassing the RCA in 14 instances, the left anterior descending (LAD) in two cases, and the circumflex artery (CX) on six occasions. There were three early deaths and one heterograft occlusion. Six-month follow-up with coronary angiography demonstrated a patency rate of 85%. This same author performed emergent CABG on two patients using this BIMA and verified the patency of both grafts with angiography at 10 and 20 days.[43] Clearly, more experience and long-term evaluation of these grafts are in order before their more generalized use can be recommended.

The Causes, Mechanisms, and Prevention of Graft Failure

From the preceding discussion, it is immediately obvious that nonautologous grafts have a limited life span when used as small arterial substitutes. Graft failure that occurs within 30 days of operation is often due to technical misadventure[45] or a hypercoagulable state. Graft failure that develops between 2 months and 2 years is often the result of intimal hyperplasia, which usually forms at the distal anastomosis[46] (Fig. 1). The progression of underlying atherosclerosis accounts for the majority of graft failures that occur beyond 2 years.[45,47]

Early Graft Failure

Technical Error

Technical errors that lead to early graft occlusion include kinking of a graft, an imperfect anastomosis, or creation of an intimal flap. In some cases, incorrect selection of an inflow or outflow vessel will result in graft failure. Early re-exploration and identification of a technical problem with correction of the defect is essential.

Hypercoagulable State

A hypercoagulable state may lead to unexplained early graft thrombosis. Prothrombotic conditions can be divided into inherited disorders and acquired or secondary disorders. The inherited disorders include antithrombin III, protein C, protein S, and fibrinolytic deficiencies. In each of these cases, there is a relative lack of one of the normally present circulating anticoagulants, predisposing the patient to intravascular thrombosis.

Although protein S and C deficiencies predispose to venous thrombosis, neither entity has been associated with primary arterial or graft occlusion. Antithrombin III deficiency has been linked to vascular graft thrombosis. Intraoperatively, the diagnosis should be entertained when heparin appears to be inadequate in preventing thrombus formation.[48] Therapy includes the administration of antithrombin III in the form of fresh frozen plasma.

The acquired coagulation disorders consist of an inhomogeneous group of abnormalities involving coagulation factors, platelets, and/or blood viscosity. Donaldson et al.[49] identified two such abnormalities—lupuslike anticoagulant and heparin-induced thrombocytopenia (HIT), as the major hypercoagulable states predisposing to graft thrombosis in the first postoperative month following infrainguinal bypass.

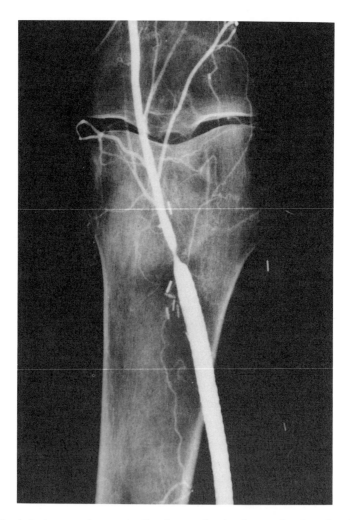

Fig. 1. Arteriogram demonstrating hyperplastic plaque that has developed at the distal anastomosis of a Dacron femoropopliteal bypass. Note the smooth tapered stenosis produced by the hyperplastic tissue. (Reprinted with permission from Loscalzo J, Creager, MA, Dzau VJ, eds. Vascular Medicine: A Textbook of Vascular Biology and Diseases. Boston, Mass., Little, Brown and Co., 1992.)

In patients previously treated with Heparin, an autoantibody that cross-reacts with Heparin and the platelet may activate platelet aggregation and thus initiate thrombosis.[50,51] Heparin-induced thrombocytopenia more frequently afflicts patients on hemodialysis because of their chronic exposure to Heparin. If vascular reconstruction must be undertaken in a patient with HIT, an alternative anticoagulant, such as Organon or Ancrod, must be used.

Lupus anticoagulant is a circulating factor that has been associated with graft thrombosis. Affected patients have an elevated partial thromboplastin time (PTT), which is paradoxically associated with an increased potential for thrombosis. Thrombosis may be averted through the perioperative administration of Heparin and Coumadin.

Preoperative recognition of coagulation disorders and appropriate perioperative therapy may prevent the occasional early graft thrombosis that is related to a hypercoagulable state.

Late Graft Failure

Intimal Hyperplasia

Multiple factors contribute to late graft failure. However, intimal hyperplasia is the leading cause of graft thrombosis that occurs within the first 2 years following arterial reconstruction. Intimal hyperplasia develops to some degree in all autogenous and synthetic grafts.[52,53] The lesion grossly appears as a white, firm, fibrous plaque impinging on the vessel lumen (Fig. 2).

Histologically, this lesion is an intimal collection of smooth muscle cells (SMC) surrounded by a matrix. Normally, smooth muscle cells native to the media have a barely detectable rate of renewal. Within 24 hours of a vascular injury, 20%–30% of medial SMC begin DNA synthesis in preparation for replication.[54,55] Smooth muscle cells migrate from the media, across the internal elastic lamina, and into the intima. These neointimal cells then continue to proliferate, producing the hyperplastic lesion.[55]

It was originally thought that intimal hyperplasia developed in response to an injury that produced endothelial denudation. Exposure of the subendothelial layer would then lead to platelet aggregation and release the platelet-derived growth factor (PDGF), a potent SMC mitogen.[56,57] PDFG would then promote SMC migration and proliferation, resulting in the development of the hyperplastic plaque.

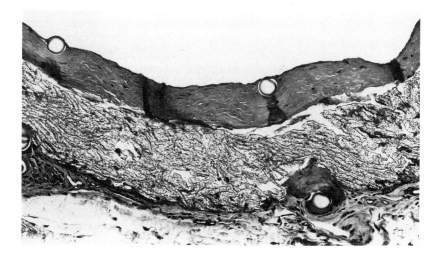

Fig. 2. Proximal anastomosis of a polytetrafluoroethylene graft (30 microns internodal distance) 60 days following implantation in the rat aorta. (Hematoxylin and eosin; 50X). A significant amount of intimal hyperplasia has developed within the graft lumen.

Recent investigations have shown that the sequence is much more complex. Endothelial cells, macrophages, and SMCs, as well as platelets, produce a variety of SMC mitogens and inhibitors. Electron microscopic studies have identified monocytes and polymorphonuclear cells on deendothelialized arterial surfaces following balloon injury.[58,59] How these various cells and growth factors interact to produce the hyperplastic response is not yet clear.

Attempts have been made to prevent and control intimal hyperplasia by a variety of pharmacological manipulations. Antiplatelet agents could, theoretically, prevent platelet aggregation and the release of the PDGF, leading to the inhibition of the hyperplastic response. Recent work has suggested that PDGF derived from platelets is only a weak stimulant of SMC proliferation.[60] This observation, combined with negative results from trials where antiplatelet agents have been used in an attempt to control intimal hyperplasia,[61,62] has led investigators to try other approaches.

The naturally occurring anticoagulant heparin has been found to allay the development of intimal hyperplasia by inhibiting SMC proliferation, migration, and matrix production.[63-66] This suppressive effect of heparin has been demonstrated in the rabbit balloon injury model[63] (Fig. 3), as well as in the vein graft model in the rat.[67] Heparin retains this effect even if it is delivered locally, avoiding the need for systemic anticoagulation.[68] Unfortunately, no clinical trials have been able to duplicate heparin's antiproliferative effect in humans.

Much attention has been focused on the effects of angiotensin-converting enzyme (ACE) inhibitors on intimal proliferation. Angiotensin II has been shown to be a potent mitogen for vascular SMC.[69] Diminishing the local production of angiotensin II in the vessel wall with ACE inhibitors might then lead to a reduction in the intimal hyperplastic response. Several studies have shown a suppression of intimal hyperplasia using the ACE inhibitor cilazapril.[70,71] Still other studies have demonstrated no small benefit following treatment with ACE inhibitors.[72-74] Recent studies in rats suggest that the combination of cilazapril and heparin is more effective in reducing intimal hyperplasia than either agent alone.[71,75] On the basis of promising experimental data, a large multicenter trial was performed to study the effects of cilazapril on the restenosis rate following coronary angioplasty. This recent randomized study failed to

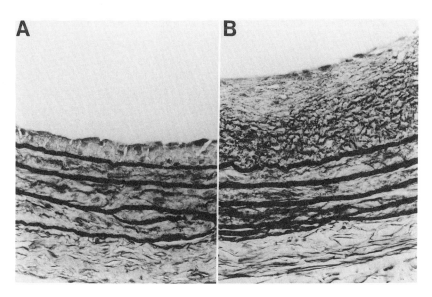

Fig. 3. Transverse section of a rat carotid artery 2 weeks after balloon injury (Verhoeff's elastic stain; 100X). (A) Treated with intravenous heparin for 14 days following the injury. (B) Control. (Reproduced with permission of Morris J. Karnovsky, M.B., B.Ch., D.Sc.)

show any advantage in the group of patients treated with ACE inhibitors.[76] There have been several hypotheses as to why this trial failed, but, unfortunately, the potential clinical use of ACE inhibition in the prevention of intimal hyperplasia is still unclear.

Modification of the inflammatory white cell response with steroids or cyclosporin might serve to prevent intimal hyperplasia. Experimental results have been conflicting. In a study using a rabbit balloon carotid injury model,[77] steroids produced a significant reduction in intimal proliferation, but in a second study in which Dacron graft was implanted in 30 animals, no difference in intimal thickness was found between steroid-treated and control animals.[78] The immunosuppressant cyclosporin has been tested in the vein graft model[79] and in the rat common iliac balloon injury model and has been shown to decrease medial thickening in both systems.[80]

Despite the multitude of promising studies in animals showing successful pharmacological manipulation of intimal hyperplasia, no drug has been shown conclusively to inhibit this process in humans.

Progression of Atherosclerotic Disease

Late graft failure occurring beyond 2 years may arise from the progression of atherosclerotic occlusive disease in the inflow or outflow vessels. Disease in the outflow tract is most common. Stenosis can develop within vein grafts after 2 years, and histologically these lesions appear to be atherosclerotic rather than hyperplastic. A recent report by Reifsnyder et al.[81] suggests that this occurrence is relatively frequent.

New Developments in the Small Vessel Bypass

In humans, endothelial cells initially proliferate and migrate onto a polymeric surface at a rate of 0.2 mm per day.[82] This migration ceases spontaneously after approximately 1 cm at each end of the graft has been covered. Plasma proteins, most prominently fibrinogen, are deposited along the remaining surface of a graft.[83] Throughout its lifespan, a prosthetic graft remains relatively thrombogenic when compared to an endothelial-lined autogenous conduit.

Despite this luminal fibrin layer, large diameter grafts have five-year patency rates of 85%–95%.[52,84] Thrombosis is prevented by the high rate of flow through these conduits. However, because of low flow rates, grafts used to bypass small vessels continue to accumulate luminal fibrin, forming an average pseudointimal thickness of 1 mm. The lumen diameter of a 6-mm graft is reduced to 4 mm by pseudo-intima, resulting in a 50% reduction in luminal area and about a 400% increase in resistance.[85] This results in a further diminution of flow through the graft, which predisposes the patient to graft thrombosis.

Attempts to design an inert prosthetic graft that does not pro-voke the coagulation cascade have been unsuccessful. An alternative would be to line a prosthetic graft with an intact, nonthrombogenic, endothelial monolayer. Two approaches have been developed to en-hance endothelial coverage of currently used prosthetic grafts. The first is to stimulate normal vascular healing through transmural or lu-minal ingrowth of endothelial cells. The second is to "seed" grafts with endothelial cells prior to implantation.

High Porosity Grafts

Golden et al.[86] have studied a high porosity (60–90 microns) PTFE graft that allows transmural migration of capillary endothelial cells into the lumen of the graft. Four weeks after implantation, the entire graft develops a confluent lining of the endothelium. Unfortu-nately, a hyperplastic SMC response often develops beneath the en-dothelial layer. Also, several reports suggest that high porosity grafts may not re-endothelialize in humans.[87,88]

Endothelial Cell Growth Factors

Numerous investigators have explored the use of endothelial cell mitogens as a stimulant of more complete and rapid endothelial cell coverage of synthetic grafts. Fibroblast growth factor (FGF) is a known potent mitogen of endothelial cells.[89] Greisler et al.[90] at-tempted to bind FGF to various biomaterials in an effort to promote endothelial coverage. They have succeeded in attaching FGF to Dac-ron and polydioxanone (PDS) grafts[90] as well as PTFE grafts.[91] Re-cently the group reported that adherence of FGF to PTFE may be improved by lining a graft with a mixture of fibrin glue containing FGF, heparin, fibrinogen, and thrombin. With this technique, there is still an initial loss of FGF from the graft following restoration of blood flow; however, FGF remained detectable for up to 30 days following graft implantation. Those PTFE grafts exposed to the fibrin glue/FGF combination demonstrated extensive capillary ingrowth and confluent endothelialization of the luminal surface as opposed to control PTFE grafts, which remained devoid of endothelium. Greisler et al.,[91] unfortunately, also found that the FGF pretreatment resulted in a thicker neointimal layer composed of myofibroblasts and collagen. It is unknown whether progression of this neointimal hyperplastic response might later jeopardize the patency of these grafts.

Endothelial Cell Seeding

Endothelial seeding of a prosthetic graft involves harvesting endothelial cells from an autogenous source, either an SV or omentum, and seeding these cells onto the luminal surface of the implanted graft. Endothelial cell seeding of prosthetic grafts has been successfully performed in dogs,[92,93] pigs,[94] and baboons.[95] Unfortunately, these favorable results have been more difficult to reproduce in humans.

A number of problems have been encountered. The lumen of the SV is normally covered with endothelial cells at a density of 1.2×105 cells/cm^2.[96] Therefore, to achieve a confluent endothelial cell layer on a prosthetic graft, a similar or greater number of endothelial cells will need to be seeded. Endothelial cell loss occurs during the harvesting procedure[97] and following the exposure of seeded grafts to flow.[98] Seeding at subconfluent densities leaves areas of the graft devoid of endothelium and prone to thrombosis. Harvested cells can be grown in tissue culture to increase the cell number. However, this may require weeks to generate an adequate yield, and the clinical situation may deteriorate in the interim.[99]

Currently used vascular prostheses have poor affinity for endothelial cells. Flowing blood creates shear forces that challenge the ability of the cell to remain adherent to the graft. Precoating of the graft with collagen,[100] Matrigel,[101] fibronectin,[101,102], and biosubstrates derived from an extracellular matrix of corneal endothelial cells have all been used.[103]

In animals, endothelial cell seeding can produce an in vivo graft completely lined with endothelial cells, and these seeded synthetic grafts have improved patency rates.[95] The endothelial cells lining these grafts are functional and release prostacyclin.[104] Platelet, as well as bacterial, adherence to seeded grafts is reduced.[105,106]

In humans, serial evaluation of seeded grafts is difficult, and there are only anecdotal reports of biopsies taken from these grafts at the time of patient death or reoperation.[107] Often follow-up is limited to noninvasive evaluation of platelet adherence to the graft surface.

Ortenwall et al.[108] examined 22 patients undergoing replacement of the infrarenal aorta with bifurcated Dacron grafts. One limb of the prosthesis was seeded, and the other served as the control. At 1, 4, and 12 months postoperatively, the seeded graft limb showed significantly less deposition of platelets compared to the control limb. These results have been reproduced in patients who had placement of seeded infrainguinal femoropopliteal bypass grafts.[109]

Recently, Magometschnigg and colleagues[99] seeded venous endothelial cells onto grafts in 13 patients requiring reoperation for peripheral vascular disease. A separate group of patients who had comparable severity of vascular disease and required femoropopliteal bypasses served as the control group. They reported early secondary patency rates of 92% for the endothelial cell seeding group and 53% for the control group. After 18 months, the amputation rate for the seeded group was 15% versus 31% in the control group.

Although evidence of the improved early patency of seeded femoropopliteal grafts in humans is beginning to accumulate,[108,110] it is less clear whether the seeding process will prevent anastomotic intimal hyperplasia and resultant late graft thrombosis. Despite years of research and over 100 studies, endothelial cell seeding continues to remain an investigational procedure.

Genetic Manipulation of Endothelial Cells

Genetic manipulation of endothelial cells is another method by which the patency of prosthetic vascular grafts might be improved. Manipulation of the cellular genome may allow the endothelial cell to produce a new protein, or the production of a protein already secreted by the cell may be increased. Retroviruses may be used to inject fragments of DNA into cells in a process called small transduction. When the host cell is infected, the cell redirects its activities toward production of the new genetic information. These genetically altered cells can then be seeded onto a prosthetic graft surface. As an example of the usefulness of this technique, cells that produce increased quantities of tissue plasminogen-activating substance or prostacylin, both antithrombotic agents normally produced by endothelial cells, might be seeded onto a prosthetic graft, reducing the potential for vascular graft thrombosis.

Endothelial cells transfected with the E. coli lacZ gene have been seeded onto prosthetic grafts implanted into the carotid artery of dogs. β-galactosidase is the protein product of the lacZ gene, and its presence in the cell cytoplasm is easily identified with an enzymic histochemical assay. Wilson et al.[111] harvested prosthetic grafts that had been previously seeded with genetically manipulated endothelial cells. Scanning electron microscopy revealed a confluent endothelial monolayer of cells attached to the graft surface that had retained their new genetic codes.

Using the lacZ gene translocation technique, Nabel et al.[112] de-endothelialized porcine iliac arteries, seeded them with altered endothelial cells, and showed that 4 weeks later the endothelium covering these denuded arteries stained positively for the protein expressed by the newly transfected gene.

Although this technique holds great promise, there are several limitations. The number of cells infected by a virus is low, so the number of cells expressing the genome is small. The size of the genetic sequence that is transfected must be less than 8,000 base pairs.[113] Larger genes cannot be introduced into the cell, nor can a large number of genetic copies be added to an individual cell. Thus, certain genes are unable to be transfected, and the amount of protein matrix that can be produced may be low.

As molecular techniques improve, gene modification may evolve as a technique that can be used to greatly enhance the patency of small diameter prosthetic grafts.

Alternatives to Current Synthetic Grafts

The search for the ultimate synthetic graft continues. Heparin has been covalently bound to PTFE grafts implanted in the carotid arteries of sheep with a successful reduction in the rate of thrombosis.[114]

A gaseous monomer may be electrically discharged onto the surface of a graft by a process called gas-flow polymerization. Grafts composed of less reactive PTFE discharged onto Dacron have been created; yet, the resulting combination seems to offer no additional clinical advantage.[115]

Polyurethane grafts are hydrophilic and may be fashioned from a wide variety of polymers. Chemical modifications alter surface properties so that platelet and leukocyte attachment is diminished.[116] Polyurethane grafts have been extensively studied in animals. Because of the wide range of polyurethane elastomers that are available, it is important that each author characterize the material that he has studied so that comparisons can be made. Acceptable patency rates and significant endothelial ingrowth have been achieved in polyurethane grafts implanted in rats.[117] Complete endothelialization and reasonable patency of fibrous polyurethane grafts in dogs has been reported.[118] Still other researchers have demonstrated poor patency rates with polyurethane grafts.[119,120] Certain polyurethanes can be enzymatically degraded by hydrogen peroxide released from leukocytes, and aneurysmal degeneration of these grafts is known to occur.[120]

Recently, Bull et al.[121] reported the results of 15 femoropopliteal reconstructions performed in humans with polyurethane grafts. There were five early occlusions, and the one-month primary patency was 66%, with a secondary patency rate of 80%.

Clearly, further laboratory evaluation and strict reporting guidelines are in order before recommendations may be made regarding the use of polyurethanes as small caliber conduits.

Conclusion

There continues to be a great need for a less thrombogenic small diameter vascular graft. The native artery is a dynamic system with constant interaction between endothelial cells, SMCs, and the circulating elements. The task of formulating a synthetic graft that closely mimics this delicate interplay is formidable. However, any progress that is made will lead to prolongation of lives and the sparing of limbs. Further advances will occur through successful interactions between cardiovascular surgeons, vascular biologists, and polymer chemists. Until then, autogenous conduits should be considered before artificial graft material is used.

References

1. Taylor LM Jr, Phinney ES, Porter JM. Present status of reversed vein bypass for lower extremity revascularization. J Vasc Surg 1986; 3(2):288–297.
2. Fogle MA, Whittemore AD, Couch NP, Mannick JA. A comparison of in situ and reversed saphenous vein grafts for infrainguinal reconstruction. J Vasc Surg 1987; 5(1):46–52.

3. Loop FD, Lytle BW, Cosgrove DM, Stewart RW, et al. Influence of the internal mammary artery graft on 10 year survival and other cardiac events. N Engl J Med 1986; 314(1):1–6.

4. Leather RP, Shah DM, Karmody AM. Infrapopliteal arterial bypass for limb salvage: increased patency and utilization of the saphenous vein used in situ. Surgery 1981; 90(6):1000–1008.

5. Veith FJ, Moss CM, Sprayregen S, Montefusco C. Preoperative saphenous venography in arterial reconstructive surgery of the lower extremity. Surgery 1979; 85(3):253–256.

6. Scales JT. Tissue reactions to synthetic materials. Proc Royal Soc Med 1953; 46(17):647–652.

7. Voorhees AB Jr, Jaretzke AL, Blakemore AH. The use of tubes constructed from Vinyon-"N" cloth in bridging arterial defects. Ann Surg 1952; 135(3):332–336.

8. Edwards WS, Lyons C. Three years experience with peripheral arterial grafts of crimped nylon and Teflon. Surg Gynecol Obstet 1958; 107(1):62–68.

9. Matsumoto H, Hasegawa T, Fuse K. A new vascular prosthesis for a small caliber artery. Surgery 1973; 74(4):519–523.

10. Campbell CD, Goldfarb D, Detton DD, et al. Expanded polytetrafluoroethylene as a small artery substitute. Trans Am Soc Artif Intern Organs 1974; 20A:86–90.

11. Campbell CD, Brooks DH, Webster MW, Bahnson HT. The use of expanded microporous polytetrafluoroethylene for limb salvage: a preliminary report. Surgery 1976; 79(5):485–491.

12. Campbell CD, Brooks DH, Webster MW, et al. Aneurysm formation in expanded polytetrafluoroethylene prostheses. Surgery 1976; 79(5):491–493.

13. Gross RE, Hurwitt ES, Bill ALH Jr, et al. Preliminary observations on the use of human arterial grafts in the treatment of certain cardiovascular defects. N Engl J Med 1948; 239(16):578–579.

14. Buckley BH, Roberts WC. Heterografts as aortocoronary bypass conduits in human beings. Am J Cardiol 1975; 36(6):823–828.

15. Tomizawa Y, Moishiki Y, Okoshi T, et al. Development of a small caliber biologic vascular graft: evaluation of its antithrombogenicity and the early healing process. ASAIO Trans 1990; 36(3):M734–737.

16. Vrandecic MO. New graft for the surgical treatment of small vessel diseases. J Cardiovasc Surg 1987; 28(6):711–714.

17. Suma H, Oku T, Sato H, et al. The Bioflow[R] experience in coronary artery bypass grafting. Tex Heart Inst J 1990; 17(2):103–105.

18. Veith FJ, Moss CM, Fell SC, et al. Expanded polytetrafluoroethylene grafts in reconstructive arterial surgery: preliminary report of the first 100 consecutive cases for limb salvage. JAMA 1978; 240(17):1867–1869.

19. Hearn AR, Charlesworth D. The early results of reconstruction of the femoral artery with a Gore-Tex prosthesis. Surgery 1979; 85(6):607–610.

20. Whittemore AD, Kent KC, Donaldson MC, et al. What is the proper role of polytetrafluoroethylene grafts in infrainguinal reconstruction: J Vasc Surg 1989; 10(3):299–305.

21. Veith FJ, Gupta SK, Ascer E, et al. Six-year prospective multicenter randomized comparison of autologous saphenous vein and expanded polytetrafluoroethylene grafts in infrainguinal arterial reconstruction. J Vasc Surg 1986; 3(1):104–114.
22. Quinones-Baldrich WJ, Busuttil RW, Baker JD, et al. Is the preferential use of polytetrafluoroethylene grafts for femoropopliteal bypass justified? J Vasc Surg 1988; 8(3):219–228.
23. Prendiville EJ, Yeager A, O'Donnell TF, et al. Long-term results with above-knee femoropopliteal expanded polytetrafluoroethylene graft. J Vasc Surg 1990; 11(4):517–524.
24. Londrey GL, Ramsey DE, Hodgson KJ, et al. Infrapopliteal bypass for severe ischemia: a comparison of autogenous vein, composite, and prosthetic grafts. J Vasc Surg 1991; 13(5):631–636.
25. Pevec WC, Darling RC, L'Italien GJ, Abbott WM. Femoropopliteal reconstruction with knitted, nonvelour Dacron versus expanded polytetrafluoroethylene. J Vasc Surg 1992; 16(1):60–65.
26. Ascer E, Veith FJ, Gupta SK, et al. Six year experience with expanded polytetrafluoroethylene arterial grafts for limb salvage. J Cardiovasc Surg 1985; 26(5):468–472.
27. Mannick JA, Maini BS. Femorofemoral grafting: indications and late results. Am J Surg 1978; 136(2):190–192.
28. Ray LI, O'Connor JB, Davis CC, et al. Axillofemoral bypass: a critical reappraisal of its role in the management of aortoiliac occlusive disease. Am J Surg 1979; 138(1):117–128.
29. Schneider JR, McDaniel MD, Walsh DB, et al. Axillofemoral bypass: outcome and hemodynamic results in high-risk patients. J Vasc Surg 1992; 15(6):952–963.
30. Keller MP, Hoch JR, Harding AD, et al. Axillopopliteal bypass for limb salvage. J Vasc Surg 1992; 15(5):817–822.
31. Rosenberg N. Dialdehyde starch tanned bovine heterografts: development. In: Sawyer PN, Kaplitt MJ, eds. Vascular Grafts. New York: Appleton-Century-Crofts, 1978: 261–270.
32. Dale WA, Lewis MR. Further experiences with bovine arterial grafts. Surgery 1976; 80(6):711–721.
33. Wagner WH, Levin PM, Treiman RL, et al. Early results of infrainguinal arterial reconstruction with a modified biological conduit. Ann Vasc Surg 1992; 6(4):325–333.
34. Cohn LH, Collins JJ. The used polytetrafluoroethylene as an aortocoronary bypass graft. In: Sawyer PN, Kaplitt MJ, eds. Vascular Grafts. New York: Appleton-Century-Crofts, 1978: 398– 403.
35. Murtra M, Mestres CA, Igual A. Long-term patency of polytetrafluoroethylene vascular grafts in coronary artery surgery. Ann Thorac Surg 1985; 39(1):86–87.
36. Yokoyama T, Gharavi MA, Lee YC, et al. Aorto-coronary artery revascularization with an expanded polytetrafluoroethylene vascular graft: a preliminary report. J Thorac Cardiovasc Surg 1978; 76(4):552–555.
37. Sapsford RN, Oakley GD, Talbot S. Early and late patency of expanded polytetrafluoroethylene vascular grafts in aorto-coronary bypass. J Thorac Cardiovasc Surg 1981; 81(6):860–864.

38. Hehrlein FW, Schlepper M, Loskot F, et al. The use of expanded poly-tetrafluoroethylene grafts for myocardial revascularization. J Cardiovasc Surg 1984; 25(6):549–553.
39. Chard RB, Johnson DC, Nunn GR, Cartmill TB. Aorto-coronary bypass grafting with polytetrafluoroethylene conduits: early and late outcome in eight patients. J Thorac Cardiovasc Surg 1987; 94(1):132–134.
40. Hartman AR, Vlay SC, Dervan JP, et al. Emergency coronary revascularization using polytetrafluoroethylene conduits in a patient in cardiogenic shock. Clin Cardiol 1991; 14(1):75–78.
41. Hancock JB, Forshaw PL, Kaye MP. Gore-Tex (polytetrafluoroethylene) in canine coronary artery bypass. J Thorac Cardiovasc Surg 1980; 80(1):94–101.
42. Sauvage LR, Schloemer R, Wood SJ, Logan G. Successful interposition synthetic graft between aorta and right coronary artery: angiographic follow-up to sixteen months. J Thorac Cardiovasc Surg 1976; 72(3):418–421.
43. Suma H, Wanibuchi Y, Terarde Y, et al. Bovine internal thoracic artery graft: successful use at urgent coronary bypass surgery. J Cardiovasc Surg 1991; 32(2):268–270.
44. Donzeau-Gouge P, Touati G, Vouhe P, et al. Coronary artery bypass grafts using bovine internal mammary artery (in French). Ann Chir Thorac Cardiovasc 1990; 40(8):599–601.
45. Whittemore AD, Clowes AW, Couch NP, Mannick JA. Secondary femoropopliteal reconstruction. Ann Surg 1981; 193(1):35–42.
46. Imparato AM, Braceo A, Kim GE, et al. Intimal and neointimal fibrous proliferation causing failure of arterial reconstruction. Surgery 1972: 72:1007–1017.
47. Wooster DL, Provan JL. Fate of the limb after failed femoropopliteal reconstruction. Can J Surg 1982;25(4):393–397.
48. Shafer AI. The hypercoagulable states. Ann Intern Med 1985; 102(6): 814–828.
49. Donaldson MC, Weinberg DS, Belkin M, et al. Screening for hypercoagulable states in vascular surgical practice: a preliminary study. J Vasc Surg 1990;11:825–831.
50. Salzman EW, Rosenberg RD, Smith MH, et al. Effect of heparin and heparin fractions on platelet aggregation. J Clin Invest 1980; 65(1):64–73.
51. King DJ, Keltin JG. Heparin-associated thrombocytopenia. Ann Intern Med 1984; 100(4):535–540.
52. Szilagyi DE, Smith RF, Elliott JP, Allen HM. Long term behavior of a Dacron arterial substitute. Ann Surg 1965; 162(3):453–477.
53. Echave V, Koornick AR, Haimov M, Jacobson JH. Intimal hyperplasia as a complication of the use of the polytetrafluoroethylene graft for femoral popliteal bypass. Surgery 1979; 86(6):791–798.
54. Clowes AW, Schwartz SM. Significance of quiescent smooth muscle cell migration in the injured rat carotid artery. Circ Res 1985; 56(1):139–145.
55. Clowes AW, Clowes MM, Fingerle J, Reidy MA. Regulation of smooth muscle cell growth in injured artery. J Cardiovasc Pharmacol 1989; 14(suppl.6):S12–S15.

56. George JN, Nurden AT, Philips DR. Molecular defects in interactions of platelets with the vessel wall. N Engl J Med 1984; 311(17):1084–1098.

57. Ross R, Glomset J, Kariya B, Harker L. A platelet-dependent serum factor that stimulates the proliferation of arterial smooth muscle cells in vitro. Proc Nat Acad Sci USA 1974; 71(4):1207–1210.

58. Lucas JF, Makhoul RG, Cole CW, et al. Mononuclear cells adhere to sites of vascular balloon catheter injury. Curr Surg 1986; 43(2):112–115.

59. Cole C, Lucas J, Mikat E, et al. Adherence of polymorphonuclear leukocytes to injured rabbit aorta. Surg Forum 1984; 440–442.

60. Jawien A, Lindner V, Bowen-Pope DF, et al. Platelet derived growth factor (PDGF) stimulates arterial smooth muscle cell proliferation in vivo. (Abstract) FASEB J 1990; 4(3):342.

61. Friedman RJ, Stemerman MB, Wenz B, et al. The effect of thrombocytopenia on experimental atherosclerotic lesion formation in rabbits: smooth muscle cell proliferation and re-endothelialization. J Clin Invest 1977; 60(5):1191–1201.

62. Radic ZS, O'Malley MK, Mikat EM, et al. The role of aspirin and dipyridamole on vascular DNA synthesis and intimal hyperplasia following de-endothelialization. J Surg Res 1986; 41(1):84–91.

63. Hoover RI, Rosenberg R, Haering W, Karnovsky MK. Inhibition of rat arterial smooth muscle cell proliferation by heparin II in vitro studies. Circ Res 1980; 47(4):578–583.

64. Majack RA, Clowes AW. Inhibition of vascular smooth muscle cell migration by heparin-like glycosaminoglycans. J Cell Physiol 1984; 118(3):253–256.

65. Snow AD, Bolender RP, Wight TN, Clowes AW. Heparin modulates the composition of the extracellular matrix domain surrounding arterial smooth muscle cells. Am J Pathol 1990; 137(2):313–330.

66. Guyton JR, Rosenberg RD, Clowes AW, Karnovsky MJ. Inhibition of rat arterial smooth muscle cell proliferation by heparin: in vivo studies with anticoagulant and nonanticoagulant heparin. Circ Res 1980; 46(5):625–634.

67. Hirsch GM, Karnovsky MJ. Inhibition of vein graft intimal proliferative lesions in the rat by heparin. Am J Pathol 1991; 139(3):581–587.

68. Edelman ER, Adams DH, Karnovsky MJ. Effect of controlled adventitial heparin delivery on smooth muscle cell proliferation following endothelial injury. Proc Nat Acad Sci USA 1990; 87(10):3773–3777.

69. Millet D, Desgranges C, Campan M, et al. Effects of angiotensions on cellular hypertrophy and c-fos expression in cultured arterial smooth muscle cells. Eur J Biochem 1992: 206(2):367–372.

70. Powell JS, Clozel JP, Muller RK, et al. Inhibitors of angiotensin-converting enzyme prevent myointimal proliferation after vascular injury. Science 1989; 245;186–188.

71. Powell JS, Muller RK, Baumgartner HR. Suppression of the vascular response to injury: the role of angiotensin-converting enzyme inhibitors. J Am Coll Cardiol 1991; 17(6 suppl. B):1378–1428.

72. Huber KC, Schwartz RS, Edwards WD, et al. Restenosis and angiotensin-converting enzyme inhibition: effects on neointimal prolifer-

ation in a porcine coronary injury model. (Abstract) Circulation 1991; 84(suppl. II):II–298.

73. Churchill DA, Seigel W, Dougherty KG, et al. Failure of enalapril to reduce coronary restenosis in a swine model. (Abstract) Circulation 1991; 84(suppl.I):II–297.

74. Lam JY, Bourassa MG, Blaine L, et al. Can cilazapril reduce the development of atherosclerotic changes in the balloon- injured porcine carotid arteries? (Abstract) Circulation 1990; 82(suppl. III):III–429.

75. Clowes AW, Clowes MM, Vergel SC, et al. Heparin and cilazapril together inhibit injury-induced intimal hyperplasia. Hypertension 1991; 18(suppl. 4):II65–II69.

76. Serruys PW, Rutsch W, Danchin N. Does the new angiotensin-converting enzyme inhibitor cilazapril prevent restenosis after percutaneous transluminal coronary angioplasty? Results of the MERCATOR study: a multicenter, European Research Trial with Cilazapril after Angioplasty to Prevent Transluminal Coronary Obstruction and Restenosis Study Group. Circulation 1992; 86(1):100–100.

77. Chervu A, Moore WS, Quinones-Baldrich WJ, Henderson T. Efficacy of corticosteroids in suppression of intimal hyperplasia. J Vasc Surg 1989; 10(2):129–134.

78. Hoepp LM, Elbadawi A, Cohn M, et al. Steroids and immunosuppression: effect on anastomotic intimal hyperplasia in femoral arterial Dacron bypass grafts. Arch Surg 1979; 114(3):273–276.

79. Saenz N, Hendren RB, Schoof DD, Folkman J. Reduction of smooth muscle hyperplasia in vein grafts in athymic rats. Lab Invest 1991; 65(1):15–22.

80. Wengrovitz M, Selassie LG, Gifford RR, Thiele BL. Cyclosporin inhibits the development of medial thickening after experimental arterial injury. J Vasc Surg 1990; 12(1):1–7.

81. Reifsnyder R, Towne JB, Seabrook GR, Blair JF, et al. Biology of long-term autogenous vein grafts: a dynamic evolution. Presented at the Program for the Society of Vascular Surgery 46th Annual Meeting; June 8–9, 1992; Chicago, Ill., p. 66.

82. Berger K, Sauvage LR, Rao AM, Wood SJ. Healing of arterial prostheses in man: its incompleteness. Ann Surg 1972; 175(1):118–127.

83. Salzman EW, Merrill EW. Interaction of blood with artificial surfaces. In: Colman RW, Hirsh J, Marder VJ, Salzman EW. Hemostasis and Thrombosis. Philadelphia, Pa.: J. B. Lippincott Co., 1982: 1335–1347.

84. DeBakey ME, Jordon GL, Abbot JP, et al. The fate of Dacron vascular grafts. Arch Surg 1964; 89:757–782.

85. Nicolaides AN. Haemodynamic and rheological aspects of vascular grafts. Acta Chir Scand Suppl 1987; 538:12–17.

86. Golden MA, Hanson SR, Kirkman TR, et al. Healing of polytetrafluoroethylene arterial grafts is influenced by graft porosity. J Vasc Surg 1990; 11(6):838–845.

87. Goldman M, McCollum CN, Hawker RJ, et al. Dacron arterial grafts: the influence of porosity, velour, and maturity on thrombogenicity. Surgery 1982; 92(6):947–952.

88. Stratton JR, Thiele BL, Ritchie JL. Natural history of platelet deposition on Dacron aortic bifurcation grafts in the first year after implantation. Am J Cardiol 1983; 52(3):371–374.

89. Lindner V, Majack RA, Reidy MA. Basic fibroblast growth factor stimulates endothelial regrowth and proliferation in denuded arteries. J Clin Invest 1990; 85(6):2004–2008.

90. Greisler HP, Klosak JJ, Dennis JW, et al. Biomaterial pretreatment with ECGF to augment endothelial cell proliferation. J Vasc Surg 1987; 5(2):393–399.

91. Greisler HP, Cziperle DJ, Kim DU, et al. Enhanced endothelializaton of expanded polytetrafluoroethylene grafts by fibroblast growth factor type I pretreatment. Surgery 1992; 112(2):244–255.

92. Herring M, Gardner A, Glover J. Seeding endothelium onto canine arterial prostheses: the effects of graft design. Arch Surg 1979; 114(6)679–682.

93. Ortenwall P, Bylock A, Kjellstrom BT, Risberg B. Seeding of ePTFE carotid interposition grafts in sheep and dogs: species-dependent results. Surgery 1988; 103(2):199–205.

94. Hollier LH, Fowl RJ, Pennell RC, et al. Are seeded endothelial cells the origin of neointima on prosthetic vascular grafts? J Vasc Surg 1986; 3(1):65–73.

95. Shepard AD, Eldrup-Jorgensen J, Keough EM, et al. Endothelial cell seeding of small caliber synthetic grafts in the baboon. Surgery 1986; 99(3):318–326.

96. Kent KC, Shindo S, Ikemoto T, Whittemore AD. Species variation and the success of endothelial cell seeding. J Vasc Surg 1989; 9(2):271–276.

97. Sharefkin JB, vanWart HE, Cruess DF, et al. Adult human endothelial cell enzymatic harvesting: estimates of efficiency and comparison of crude and partially purified bacterial collagenase preparations by replicate microwell culture and fibronectin degradation measured by enzyme-linked immunosorbent assay. J Vasc Surg 1986; 4(6):567–577.

98. Rosenman JE, Kempczinski RF, Pearce WH, Silberstein EB. Kinetics of endothelial cell seeding. J Vasc Surg 1985; 2(6):778–784.

99. Magometschnigg H, Kadletz M, Vodrazka M, et al. Prospective clinical study with in vitro endothelial cell lining of expanded polytetrafluoroethylene grafts in crural repeat reconstruction. J Vasc Surg 1992; 15(3)527–535.

100. Williams SK, Schneider T, Kapelan B, Jarrell BE. Formation of a functional endothelium on vascular grafts. J Electron Microsc Tech 1991; 19(4):439–451.

101. Patterson RB, Keller JD, Silberstein EB, Kempczinski RF. A comparison between fibronectin and Matrigel pretreated ePTFE vascular grafts. Ann Vasc Surg 1989; 3(2):160–166.

102. Seeger JM, Klingman N. Improved endothelial cell seeding with cultured cells and fibronectin-coated grafts. J Surg Res 1985; 38(6):641–647.

103. Schneider A, Melmed RN, Schwall H, et al. An improved method for endothelial cell seeding on polytetrafluoroethylene small caliber vascular grafts. J Vasc Surg 1992; 15(4):649–656.

104. Sharp WV, Schmidt SP, Donovan DL. Prostaglandin biochemistry of seeded endothelial cells on Dacron prostheses. J Vasc Surg 1986; 3(2):256–264.
105. Sharefkin JB, Latker C, Smith M, et al. Early normalization of platelet survival by endothelial seeding of Dacron arterial prostheses in dogs. Surgery 1982; 92(2)385–393.
106. Rosenman JE, Kempczinski RF, Berlatzky Y, et al. Bacterial adherence to endothelial-seeded polytetrafluoroethylene grafts. Surgery 1985; 98(4):816–823.
107. Herring M, Baughman S, Glover J. Endothelium develops on seeded human arterial prosthesis: a brief clinical note. J Vasc Surg 1985; 2(5):727–730.
108. Ortenwall P, Wadenvike H, Kutti J, Risberg B. Endothelial cell seeding reduces thrombogenicity of Dacron grafts in humans. J Vasc Surg 1990; 11(3):403–410.
109. Deutsch M, Fischlein T, Eberl T, et al. Human in vitro endothelialization of ePTFE vascular graft: an initial clinical report (Abstract). Presented at the International Society for Cardiovascular Surgery Scientific Program; June 1990; Los Angeles, Calif., p. 30.
110. Herring MB, Compton RS, LeGrand DR, et al. Endothelial seeding of polytetrafluoroethylene popliteal bypasses: a preliminary report. J Vasc Surg 1987; 6(2):114–118.
111. Wilson JM, Birinyi KL, Salomon RN, et al. Implantation of vascular grafts lined with genetically modified endothelial cells. Science 1989; 244:1344–1346.
112. Nabel EG, Plautz G, Boyce FM, et al. Recombinant gene expression in vivo within endothelial cells of the arterial wall. Science 1989; 244:1342–1344.
113. Stanley JC, Podrazik RM, Messina LM. Therapeutic potential of genetic engineering on vascular disease. In: Yao JST, Pearce WH, eds. Vascular Surgery. Philadelphia, Pa.: W. B. Saunders, 1992: 64.
114. Esquivel CO, Bjork CG, Bergentz SE, et al. Reduced thrombogenic characteristics of expanded polytetrafluoroethylene and polyurethane arterial grafts after heparin bonding. Surgery 1984; 95(1):102–107.
115. Greisler HP, Dennis JW, Schwarcz TH, et al. Plasma polymerized tetrafluorethylene/polyethylene terephthalate vascular prostheses. Arch Surg 1989; 124(8):967–972.
116. Kambic HE. Polyurethane small artery substitutes. ASAIO Trans 1988; 34(4):1047–1050.
117. Hess F, Jerusalem C, Braun B. The endothelialization process of a fibrous polyurethane microvascular prosthesis after implantation in the abdominal aorta of the rat: a scanning electron microscopic study. J Cardiovasc Surg 1983; 24(5):516–524.
118. Hess F, Braun B, Jersualem C, et al. Endothelialization of polyurethane vascular prostheses implanted in the dog carotid and femoral artery. J Cardiovasc Surg 1988; 29(4):458–463.
119. Martz H, Paynter R, Forest JC, et al. Microporous hydrophilic polyurethane vascular grafts as substitutes in the abdominal aorta of dogs. Biomaterials 1987; 8(1):3–11.

120. Brothers TE, Stanley JC, Burket WE, Graham LM. Small-caliber poly-urethane and polytetrafluoroethylene grafts: a comparative study in a canine aortoiliac model. J Biomed Mater Res 1990; 24(6):761–771.
121. Bull PG, Denck H, Guidoin R, Gruber H. Preliminary clinical experi-ence with polyurethane vascular prostheses in femoropopliteal recon-struction. Eur J Vasc Surg 1992; 6(2):217–224.

Index

Alternative bypass methods
  arterial conduits in, 47–108
  internal mammary artery usage
    in, 111–163
  saphenous vein usage in,
    167–225
  venous conduits in, 29–44
Angioplasty
  balloon, intraoperative, 267–278
  laser, intraoperative, 279–286
  patch. *See* Patching techniques
Angiotensin-converting enzyme,
    inhibitors preventing intimal
    hyperplasia, 301–302
Aortic disease
  innominate artery-coronary ar-
    tery venous bypass in,
    185–189
  "no-touch" technique in, 151,
    154, 185, 188
  right gastroepiploic artery in,
    60, 241
Arm vein grafts, 33–37
  clinical results of, 34, 36
  indications for, 33–35
  patency compared to internal
    mammary artery and saphe-
    nous vein grafts, 34
  pathophysiology of occlusion in,
    35–36
Artificial grafts. *See* Prosthetic vas-
    cular grafts
Atherosclerosis
  aortic
    and management of debris in
      crossclamped diseased aorta,
      174, 241–243

    "no-touch" technique in, 60,
      150–151, 154, 185, 188, 241
  coronary endarterectomy in,
    251–253
  resistance to
    in internal mammary artery,
      7–8, 74, 111, 135, 141, 145
    in lateral costal artery, 105
    in right gastroepiploic artery, 68
    in saphenous vein grafts, 20–21
    in splenic artery, 92
Atrial fistula creation for anastomo-
    sis to sequential vein graft,
    217–225
  clinical experience with, 218
  experimental work in, 218–224
  size of fistula affecting, 219–224

Balloon angioplasty, intraoperative,
    267–278
  case reports of, 273–276
  results of, 268–269, 272–273
  technique in, 272
  types of lesions in, 270–271
Basilic vein. *See* Arm vein grafts
Bilateral internal mammary artery
    grafts, 111–123
Biological grafts. *See* Prosthetic vas-
    cular grafts
Bridge grafts, 167, 169

Calcium channel blockers prevent-
    ing arterial spasm, 80, 87
Cephalic vein. *See* Arm vein grafts
Coagulation disorders, and failure
    of prosthetic vascular grafts,
    297–299

317